Clinical Intuition in Psychotherapy

The Norton Series on Interpersonal Neurobiology
Allan N. Schore, PhD, Series Editor
Daniel J. Siegel, MD, Founding Editor

The field of mental health is in a tremendously exciting period of growth and conceptual reorganization. Independent findings from a variety of scientific endeavors are converging in an interdisciplinary view of the mind and mental well-being. An interpersonal neurobiology of human development enables us to understand that the structure and function of the mind and brain are shaped by experiences, especially those involving emotional relationships.

The Norton Series on Interpersonal Neurobiology will provide cutting-edge, multidisciplinary views that further our understanding of the complex neurobiology of the human mind. By drawing on a wide range of traditionally independent fields of research—such as neurobiology, genetics, memory, attachment, complex systems, anthropology, and evolutionary psychology—these texts will offer mental health professionals a review and synthesis of scientific findings often inaccessible to clinicians. These books aim to advance our understanding of human experience by finding the unity of knowledge, or consilience, that emerges with the translation of findings from numerous domains of study into a common language and conceptual framework. The series will integrate the best of modern science with the healing art of psychotherapy.

A NORTON PROFESSIONAL BOOK

Clinical Intuition in Psychotherapy

The Neurobiology of Embodied Response

Terry Marks-Tarlow

Foreword by Allan N. Schore

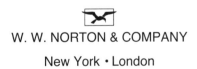

W. W. NORTON & COMPANY

New York • London

Epigraphs reprinted by permission of Albella Arthur, University of California Press, Grand Central Publishing, HarperCollins Publishers, and Hand to Hand Publishing.

For information about permission to reproduce selections from this book, write to Permissions, W. W. Norton & Company, Inc., 500 Fifth Avenue, New York, NY 10110

For information about special discounts for bulk purchases, please contact W. W. Norton
Special Sales at specialsales@wwnorton.com or 800-233-4830

Manufacturing by Quad Graphics, Fairfield
Book design by Midatlantic Publishing Services, Baltimore, MD
Production manager: Leeann Graham

Library of Congress Cataloging-in-Publication Data

Marks-Tarlow, Terry, 1955-
 Clinical intuition in psychotherapy : the neurobiology of embodied response / Terry Marks-Tarlow.—1st ed.
     p. cm. -- (The Norton series on interpersonal neurobiology) (A Norton professional book)
 Includes bibliographical references and index.
 ISBN 978-0-393-70703-8 (hardcover)
 1. Intuition. 2. Neurobiology. 3. Psychotherapy. I. Title.
 BF315.5.M375 2012
 616.89'14--dc23
                              2011052852

ISBN: 978-0-393-70703-8

W. W. Norton & Company, Inc., 500 Fifth Avenue, New York, N.Y. 10110
                         www.wwnorton.com
W. W. Norton & Company Ltd., Castle House, 75/76 Wells Street, London W1T 3QT

1 2 3 4 5 6 7 8 9 0

To all psychotherapists—past, present, and future—

to honor your internal gifts.

Contents

Acknowledgments

This book could never have been written without the ceaseless support and inspiration of my loving husband, Buzz, and two beautiful children, Cody and Darby. Beyond my family and Topanga community, I heartily thank each and every patient who graces my life and these pages for endless opportunities to learn and grow along with them. I am indebted to Allan Schore, the current editor of W. W. Norton's Interpersonal Neurobiology series, for his encouragement, mentorship, and wise guidance. I thank Deborah Malmud at Norton for readily embracing the topic of clinical intuition and for her impeccable eye as an editor, as well as to Libby Burton, Vani Kannan, and Ben Yarling for careful editorial assistance. My gratitude goes to Sandy Halperin for her boundless enthusiasm and involvement in all stages of this project and to Tely Toumani for the time, care, and detailed feedback she poured into early drafts of the manuscript. Thanks to Beth Lutz for reading a draft and contributing a clinical vignette, to Karin Hart for being an attentive reader, and to Jennifer Franklin, Michael Summerlin, Sherry Bronow, and Darlene D'Arezio for friendship and support during the creation of this book. Finally, my hearty appreciation extends to all friends and colleagues who contributed visual images: Tom Arizmendi, Remy Ashe, Jan Berlin, Günther Bernatzky, Pixie Brown, Margaret Bryant, Georgianne Cowan, Gene Blevins, Victoria Davis, Jean Decety, Scott Eberle, Lesleigh Gasbarre, Oliver Gaspirtz, Jaclyn Gisburne, Jeanne Heileman, Jon Hurd, Karen Makoff, Jaak Panksepp, Benedicte Schoyen, Richard Taylor, Norman Thrower, Susan Trien, and Victor Yalom.

Foreword

by Allan N. Schore

It's my pleasure to introduce the reader to the creative mind of Terry Marks-Tarlow. Psychotherapists are now extremely interested in clinical models that focus upon the implicit affective communications transmitted "beneath the words" of the therapeutic alliance. At the same time, mental health workers of all professions and schools are now asking, in a practical sense, how does current neuroscience inform and even alter the way we work with patients, especially patients with early attachment trauma?

The attempt to throw new light on the deeper mechanisms of psychotherapy is a daunting challenge, but right at the start, let me say that in the following chapters the author succeeds. In this important contribution Marks-Tarlow puts under a psychological microscope the rapid "invisible" right brain-to-right brain communications that are rapidly expressed beneath the conscious awareness of both members of the therapeutic dyad, yet are fundamental to the change process of psychotherapy. She argues that this interpersonal neurobiological perspective actually changes the way we work. In fact at a number of points in this groundbreaking book the author describes the paradigm shift that is occurring in psychotherapy. Before I begin to describe in detail how I believe this book offers an important contribution to the paradigm shift, I'd like to place this work in a larger context.

In a number of contributions over the last 10 years I have argued that the field of psychotherapy (and indeed all clinical and experimental life sciences) is now undergoing a transformation, a true paradigm shift. The ongoing explosion of brain research, especially in affective, developmental, and social neuroscience, is now being rapidly absorbed into updated psychological models of clinical practice. This accelerating interdisciplinary trend towards the integration of the psychological and biological realms is transforming the mental health field. Indeed, this paradigm shift is generating a fresh approach and deeper understanding of both the developmental psychopathological origins of the emotional deficits that lie at the core of psychiatric disorders as well as the psychodynamics and neurodynamics of the change processes embedded within psychotherapy.

In my most recent book *The Science of the Art of Psychotherapy* (also published in this Norton Series on Interpersonal Neurobiology), I offer a chapter entitled "Toward a New Paradigm of Psychotherapy" (Schore, 2012). In that work I look back to propose that the psychological and psychiatric disciplines have witnessed a transformation from the behavioral psychology of the 1960s and 1970s to the dominance of the cognitive paradigm that arose in the 1970s and 1980s. This shift in theoretical perspective altered our models of psychopathology and psychotherapy, from a period which generated psychological models of psychotherapeutically changing the patient's maladaptive *behavior* to a period when science was observing not only external behavior but also internal *cognitive* processes (e.g., memory, attention, perception, representational schemas, consciousness, narratives, and language). And so, in the last quarter of the century, we entered into a period of dominance of a cognitive paradigm and a directly related cognitive psychology. The fundamental principle in this paradigm was to change the patient's maladaptive conscious *cognitions*, and this was expressed in the creation of cognitive-behavioral forms of therapy.

More recently the "decade of the brain," the period from the mid-nineties to the middle of the 2000s, acted as the next transformational force, thrusting bodily-based *emotions and psychobiological states* into the center of both research and clinical models. Although mostly ignored in previous eras, for the first time science increasingly focused its methodologies and burgeoning technologies directly upon the problem of emotion. A large number of clinicians turned their attention to these discoveries of the neurobiological mechanisms of emotion, looking for the practical applications in their work with patients. Psychotherapists have long been interested in development, but now the shift was from cognitive to emotional development. Essential emotional functions are dominant in the earliest periods of human development, and for the rest of the life span these rapid-acting psychobiological processes operate at levels beneath explicit conscious awareness, thereby reflecting implicit mind body processes. Thus the current paradigm shift from behavior and cognition to emotion has acted as a major force in resolving the Cartesian problem and generating more powerful theoretical models that integrate biology and psychology, "nature and nurture."

This quantitative surge in clinically relevant research as well as the qualitative shift in our theoretical constructs has greatly expanded our models of the central role of emotions in developmental, psychopathological, and psychotherapeutic processes. The current rich dialogue between scientists and clinicians has converged on the centrality of adaptive implicit (unconscious) bodily-based affective processes in the human experience, and has contributed to the paradigm shift from conscious cognition to unconscious affect. Indeed I have suggested that the early developing right brain hemisphere, "the emotional brain," "the social brain," and not the later maturing linguistic left brain is dominant in the human experience, and that the most fundamental problems of human existence cannot be understood without addressing this primal realm (Schore, 1994, 2003a, 2003b, 2012).

Over the last two decades a central theme of my own studies in developmental affective neuroscience and developmental neuropsychoanalysis has dictated that the right hemisphere, the biological substrate of the human unconscious, is not only dominant in infancy but over all stages of the life cycle. In 2003, in *Affect Dysregulation and the Repair of the Self,* I put forth the argument that the implicit, nonconscious survival functions of the right, and not the language functions of the left, are dominant in development and in psychotherapy. In subsequent writings I described how not only survival but also the most complex highest human functions—stress regulation, intersubjectivity, humor, empathy, compassion, morality, creativity, and intuition—are all right brain functions. I also suggested that an expanded capacity for right- and not left-brain processing lies at the core of clinical expertise. Much of the therapist's knowledge that accumulates with clinical experience is implicit, operates at rapid unconscious levels beneath levels of awareness, and is expressed as clinical intuition. This implicit relational knowledge is nonverbally communicated in rightbrain–to–right brain affective transactions that lie beneath the words within the therapeutic alliance.

Expanding upon these ideas in 2008, Judith and I described the rapid, implicit right brain/mind/body affective transactions that occur within patient–therapist transference–countertransference communications:

> In this intersubjective dialogue, the psychobiologically attuned, *intuitive* clinician, from the first point of contact, is learning the nonverbal moment-to-moment rhythmic structures of the client's internal states, and is relatively flexibly and fluidly modifying her own behavior to synchronize with that structure, thereby co-creating with the client a growth-facilitating context for the organization of the therapeutic alliance. (J. Schore & A. Schore, 2008, p. 16)

This interpersonal neurobiological perspective resonated with earlier clinical observations that the therapist's capacity for intersubjective communication within the psychotherapeutic relationship depends upon her "being open to *intuitive* sensing of what is happening in the back of the patient's words and, often, back of his conscious awareness" (Bugental, 1987, p. 11), and that "The analyst, by means of reverie and *intuition*, listens with the right brain directly to the analysand's right brain" (Marcus, 1997, p. 238)

At a number of points in this groundbreaking book Terry Marks-Tarlow also describes the paradigm shift that is occurring in psychotherapy. Indeed, she makes an important contribution to the shift by utilizing a creative interpersonal neurobiological lens to bring into focus a clinical process that has long been appreciated, if not understood, by practicing clinicians—intuition. Right at the outset she boldly states, "First, clinical intuition fills the gaps between theory and practice. Second, clinical intuition involves the perception of relational patterns, both in self and other. Third, clinical intuition is a necessary ingredient for deep change during psychotherapy." (p. 3). Furthermore she asserts, "The function of intuition is to allow novel information that arises from moment-to-moment shifts in the emotional contours of the therapeutic relationship" (p. 19).

In the body of this remarkable volume the author launches into a deep exploration of the right brain implicit process of intuition in a variety of adaptive functions that are fundamental to the change process of psychotherapy: empathy, play, humor, imagination, development, and wisdom. The journey inward into the deeper strata of human consciousness is described in not only the experience-near language of subjectivity and metaphor but also in evocative visual images, many created by the author. In addition to being a gifted clinician with decades of experience, Marks-Tarlow has also published in the nonlinear dynamic sciences and has written very well-received contributions to the science of play behavior. The tone of this book, however, is not at all technical. Indeed it's almost playful, light, and familiar, and yet she offers the reader, in a very compelling and comprehensible fashion, a large body of complex, clinically-relevant interdisciplinary neurobiological and psychobiological information. Importantly, by using the psychobiological lens of regulation theory (Schore & Schore, 2008) she translates the meaning of the research for clinical practice. Side-by-side with objective scientific data she describes in right brain metaphorical language and images the subtle intersubjective affective moments of engagement and disengagement, of rupture and repair between her subjectivity and the patient's subjectivity. Frequently she documents not only her countertransferential psychological but physiological intuitive responses to her patient's implicit affective communications.

In ongoing discussions and many fascinating case examples Marks-Tarlow highlights the essential role of clinical intuition in psychotherapy, especially focusing on the unconscious, implicit processing of emotion. In light of the current paradigm shift from conscious cognition to unconscious affect she states, "Precisely because clinical intuition operates on implicit levels, we are just as likely to resonate with dissociated emotion as we are to resonate with that which is fully embodied into conscious awareness" (p. 23). Throughout the book she offers numerous clinical vignettes of spontaneous right-brain nonverbal emotional communications between herself and her patients that lie beneath their words. In tandem, the author also cites a significant amount of very recent neuroscience research that support her clinical models of intuition. On that matter I refer the reader to recent comprehensive reviews, which clearly establish the central role of the right brain in the unconscious processing of emotion (e.g., Gainotti, 2012; McGilchrist, 2009; Schore, 2003a, 2003b, 2012).

This book is a prime example of how recent advances in neuroscience are altering our conceptions of the mechanisms by which psychotherapy alters mind, brain, and body at both conscious and especially unconscious levels. The current paradigm shift from cognition to emotion is paralleled by a shift from the left hemisphere to the right hemisphere. We can no longer think of "the brain" as two halves of a single entity. Rather, these two systems process different types of information in very different ways. Numerous studies now indicate that the right and left human brain hemispheres differ in macrostructure, ultrastructure, physiology, chemistry, and control of behavior. Indeed, the left hemisphere of the vertebrate brain is specialized for the control of well-established patterns of behavior under ordinary and familiar circumstances. In contrast, the right hemisphere is the primary seat of emotional arousal and, as explicated in this book, the processing of *novel information*. There is now agreement that verbal, conscious, rational, and serial information processing takes place in the left brain hemisphere, "the left mind," whereas nonverbal, unconscious, holistic intuitive processing of emotional information takes place in the right brain hemisphere, "the right mind."

Supporting Marks-Tarlow's theses, in my own work on the primacy of right brain affective intuitive process in psychotherapy (J. Schore & A. Schore, 2008; A. Schore, 2011, 2012) I have noted that the definition of intuition, "the ability to understand or know something immediately, without conscious reasoning" (*Compact Oxford English Dictionary of Current English*, 2005) clearly implies right- and not left-brain processing. Psychological theoreticians now assert that intuition depends on accessing large banks of implicit knowledge formed from unarticulated person–environment exchanges that occur between environmental input and the individual's phenomenological experience (Narvaez, 2010). Intuition is being defined as "the subjective experience associated with the use of knowledge gained through implicit learning" (Lieberman, 2000, p. 109). The description of intuition as "direct knowing that seeps into conscious awareness without the conscious mediation of logic or rational process" (Boucouvalas, 1997, p. 7) describes a right- and not a left-brain function.

Writing in the psychoanalytic literature, Dorpat (2001) observes, "Intuitions, images, and emotions derived chiefly from the primary process system provide an immediate and prereflective awareness of our vital relations with both ourselves and others" (p. 450).

In the neuroscience literature, Volz and von Cramon (2006) conclude that intuition is related to the unconscious, is derived from stored nonverbal representations—such as images, feelings, physical sensations, and metaphors—and is "often reliably accurate." Intuition is expressed not in literal language but is "embodied" in a "gut feeling" or in an initial guess that subsequently biases our thought and inquiry. "The gist information is realized on the basis of the observer's implicit knowledge rather than being consciously extracted on the basis of the observer's explicit knowledge" (p. 2084). Other models of intuition generated by neuroscience are highlighting the adaptive capacity of "embodied cognition." Allman et al. (2005) assert, "We experience the intuitive process at a visceral level. Intuitive decision-making enables us to react quickly in situations that involve a high degree of uncertainty which commonly involve social interactions" (p. 370). These researchers demonstrate that right prefrontal-insula and anterior cingulate relay a fast intuitive assessment of complex social situations in order to allow the rapid adjustment of behavior in quickly changing and therefore uncertain social situations. Expanding upon this, I have suggested that intuitive processing is generated in the subcortical-cortical vertical axis of the therapist's (and patient's) right brain, from the right amygdala, right insula, and right anterior cingulate to the right orbitofrontal system (Schore, 2011).

In my clinical writings I have also described the important role of clinical intuition in an enactment, a particularly stressful but potentially growth facilitating affective experience within the therapeutic alliance. These transference–countertransference ruptures of the therapeutic relationship, often associated with relational trauma, are characterized by a density of negative affect and a high degree of uncertainty on both sides of the dyad. The right brain–to–right brain mechanism that is accessed for the negotiation of this "collision of subjectivities" (Bromberg, 2011) is essentially the same process that developmentalists call "disruption and repair" or "interactive repair" following a dyadic misattunement. In order to optimally navigate through the relational uncertainty of an enactment, the therapist must remain psychobiologically attuned to the patient in a state of right brain–to–right brain connection and at the same time access an intuitive fast, emotional, and effortless right brain decision process (Schore, 2011, 2012).

In a number of highly evocative clinical examples Marks-Tarlow confirms this model by documenting, in some detail, how the therapist's moment-to-moment negotiation of intersubjective rupture and repair within these problematic heightened affective moments occurs not by explicit, linear verbal secondary process cognition, but by implicit, nonlinear, non-verbal primary process clinical intuition. In line with her proposal that clinical intuition is a necessary ingredient for deep psychotherapeutic change, she describes clinical exchanges demonstrating that unlike the patient's earlier experiences, a co-constructed relational repair process allows him or her to cope with stressful states of negatively charged affect arousal as well as novel intersubjective contexts. Over time, these interactively regulated experiences enhance right brain affective functions and are expressed in a developmental advance in self-regulation. A central theme that emerges over the rich variety of cases across all the chapters is that the clinician's use of right brain intuitive over left brain rational interpretative approaches is a central mechanism of the psychotherapy change mechanism.

Although the essential therapeutic process of clinical intuition applies across all forms of psychotherapy, Marks-Tarlow clearly demonstrates the clinical effectiveness of a neurobiologically-informed, affectively focused psychodynamic approach, especially in cases dealing with early relational attachment trauma that has blocked emotional growth. Shedler (2010) cites empirical evidence to show that as opposed to cognitive therapies, "psychodynamic therapy sets in motion psychological processes that lead to ongoing change, even after therapy has ended" (p. 101), and that beyond symptom remission, "psychodynamic therapy may foster inner resources and capacities that allow richer, freer, and more fulfilling lives" (p. 107). Indeed this book compellingly argues that the implicit mechanisms by which the disciplined use of the therapist's intuitive, spontaneous right brain functions can not only alleviate the patient's affect-dysregulating symptomatology, but also facilitate the growth of the most complex human abilities, the adaptive self-regulating functions of not the rational but the emotional brain.

Throughout the upcoming chapters the author's creativity is expressed in her ability to verbally and nonverbally capture the essential events that occur at an implicit level within the therapeutic dyad: the rapid yet highly significant affective shifts in intersubjectivity, and the realignment of the therapist's embodied subjectivity with the patient's embodied subjectivity, at unconscious and then conscious levels. Along the way the inner searchlight of her intense curiosity focuses upon numerous phenomena that have heretofore seemed to be tangential to psychotherapy—clinical intuition, play, humor, imagination, and wisdom. Seamlessly integrating eastern and western psychology, implicit affective clinical data, and neuroscience research, mind and body, she makes a compelling case that these background right brain processes that operate beneath the horizon of conscious awareness lie not only at the core of the psychotherapy change process, but at the heart of human experience. Reader, both your left and right brains are in for an intellectual and emotional treat.

Clinical Intuition in Psychotherapy

Introduction

As a graduate student in clinical psychology at UCLA during the late 1970s and early 1980s, I spent a year sitting in classrooms studying theories about personality, development, psychopathology, and treatment in psychotherapy. In this heavily academic program, I did not get near a patient until my second year. The ivory tower assumption was that lots of theory would aid in the empirical study as well as practice of our trade. This approach contrasted sharply with my paraprofessional roots at the Southern California Counseling Center where I supervised shortly after licensure. Located in a rough neighborhood of Los Angeles, the center served a clientele that was embroiled in drugs, gangs, poverty, and trauma. The humanistic assumption was that empathic people, through their very humanness, were equipped to counsel others who were struggling with similar issues in life. At first I was amazed that practitioners with the least amount of training were paired with clients who harbored the greatest problems and symptoms. Yet, to my surprise, even for counselors who lacked much formal training, under the guidance of strong supervision things usually worked out.

Over the years I have wrestled with these opposite philosophies and approaches to psychotherapy. Historically, I have taken refuge in theory, outside resources, and the authority of others. As a child, I did not trust my body's instincts as a source of moment-to-moment guidance. This problem has plagued me throughout life. In my early forays into drawing, I copied the world as it appeared exactly, not believing I could craft an image from the inner eye of imagination. As a rock climber, I froze every time I tried to lead a climb, even on easy routes that I could scale effortlessly when following my partner. Over and over, I have trusted outer authorities more than my own inner counsel.

Upon entering my first clinical practicum, during my second year of graduate school, I recall the period just before seeing my first patient. I spent weeks churning and worrying, trying to figure out how the session would go. Over and over I asked myself the same questions.

How should I greet him?

What should I say?

How can I be of help?

Will he want to come back?

When that fateful day finally came, my actual experience was nothing like what I had envisioned. My first patient and I launched into places I could not have imagined on my own. The relationship took on a life of its own. This was my first taste of intersubjectivity, where what takes place in the space between two people has the momentum to carry both along. In contrast to my questions and self-doubts, somehow I knew *exactly* what to say in the moment of the encounter. All that fretting had been wasted energy.

Since that first session and with many subsequent ones under my belt, slowly I have come to trust in the wisdom of embodied experience. After 30 years of clinical practice, I directly sense my fullest contribution to others when I am in the flow and fluctuations of body-driven intuition. I also sense that patients are most open to my contributions to their healing and growth when they achieve similar states. The writing of this book arose from these early origins plus inner and outer journeys since.

My first book (Marks-Tarlow, 1996) was a creativity curriculum for teachers, emerging after I finally admitted to myself I was more interested in self-expression than in psychopathology. While fascinated with the creative process in others, I was not yet ready to dive in fully myself and so I wrote about it instead. My last book, *Psyche's Veil: Psychotherapy, Fractals and Complexity*, represented a leap into the creative void. After studying nonlinear science for more than a decade, I produced a case-based book blending contemporary holistic science with clinical practice.

The current book integrates my multiple passions still further. My interest in nonlinear science is tucked inside these pages, since deep transformation of all kinds is nonlinear. Within psychotherapy true change emerges unpredictably, on its own timetable, in full context. Its course cannot be mapped out with theory or planned systematically in a step-by-step fashion. This is precisely why intuition is so central to the clinical process. My interest in creativity appears in the current book as well. The working of intuition is inherently creative. Change involves traveling somewhere new. As therapists we must be as up for the journey as our patients are. Our willingness to embrace novelty both models and inspires the courage necessary to break beyond the bounds of what we already know and do. While books, reason, conscious strategy, and other workings of the left-brain have their place, this book highlights right-brain awareness of clinical intuition as the source of overall coordination, change, guidance, and agency during clinical practice.

Chapter 1 offers a taste of the book as a whole. Clinical intuition is defined from a neurobiological perspective as a right-brain, fully embodied mode of perceiving, relating, and responding to the ongoing flows and changing dynamics of psychotherapy. As clinical intuition picks up on interpersonal nuance, it draws upon immediate sensory, emotional and imaginal data. Three threads run through this book. First, clinical intuition fills the gap between theory and practice. Second, clinical intuition involves the perception of relational patterns, both in self and other. Third, clinical intuition is a necessary ingredient for deep change during psychotherapy. Brief clinical examples are designed to bring the material alive. In general, some case studies found throughout this book are composites, although many are real cases written with patient permission and fictionalized dialogue.

Chapter 2 examines how the body "has a mind of its own" in the form of *implicit processes* at the foundation of clinical intuition. In contrast to explicit processes at the basis of language, thought, and cognitive learning, implicit processes drive emotional learning, form the bedrock of relational patterns, and serve as the affective core for a sense of self. During psychotherapy, explicit learning requires conscious, deliberate efforts to think, strategize, and make decisions. By contrast, implicit learning operates beneath conscious awareness in automatic, immediate, and effortless ways. In the heat of a clinical encounter, we continually shuttle between these two modes. Intuition provides the raw data for conscious deliberation to follow up, seek feedback, and evaluate. A detailed clinical case illustrates how clinical intuition unwittingly targets the emotionally charged *zone between implicit and explicit* levels—the space between conscious and unconscious processes that is often most ripe for change.

Chapter 3 uncovers implicit roots of clinical intuition within human empathy, as well as roots of human empathy within the limbic circuitry of the care system as shared by all mammals. Impulses to nurture and bond with children, other relatives, and community members provide the natural motivation to understand the emotions of others and to penetrate their minds. I offer a tale of animal intuition to illustrate the power of this mammalian instinct, which serves as a prelude to discuss the neurobiology of empathy. A case demonstrates how clinical intuition helped to restore the natural empathic bond between a mother with severe early abuse and her newborn baby.

Chapter 4 introduces the importance of play to clinical intuition. As children develop, they discover new ways to be, think, feel, and relate to

others through play. Along with the care system, play is part of the instinctual repertoire of all mammals, helping to socialize animals into group
living. In humans, along with socialization, play serves to ground the developing self within its unique subjectivity. During psychotherapy, play
emerges spontaneously amid trust and full engagement. Clinical examples highlight how play during psychotherapy helps to broaden positive
emotion, increase intrinsic motivation, instill personal agency, and expand affect tolerance.

Chapter 5 explores how play within clinical intuition often takes the
form of humor. All therapists have a unique sense of humor that affectively colors their interventions. To utilize and receive humor taps into
idiosyncratic language that is unique to each patient. Humor arises from
the relational unconscious as it points toward the *quality* of the therapeutic relationship, indicating its implicit emotional flows, relational defenses, and potential blocks to change. Whether initiated by the patient or
therapist, humor represents an invitation to communicative play, opening
up the potential for new realms of mutual bonding and exploration. But
like any other powerful tool, humor can be abused if used in service of
avoidance, numbing, dissociation, or humiliation. Clinical examples reveal positive uses of humor to buffer pain to within tolerable limits and to
provide a safety net to approach shameful topics.

Chapter 6 explores the play of imagination within clinical intuition. Intuition not only taps into things as they already are—how patients feel
and see the world plus how this perspective gets reflected in transfer-
ence/countertransference dynamics in the room—but it also taps into
how things might be—how people might heal and grow and how we
might help them do so. Whether arising in the therapist or in the patient,
imagination often takes the form of spontaneous imagery that is sensory-
based and appears as sounds, pictures, or bodily sensations. Such imagery
represents the highest form of metaphor making by the right brain, where
past experience, present circumstances, and future imaginings are compared by noting similarities and differences. A detailed case reveals how
patient-generated imagery can serve as an embodied metaphor, leading to
deeper insight about underlying emotions and relational truths than
words alone.

Chapter 7 examines developmental foundations for intuition. Just as
rats need to explore a physical space from all angles, so, too, must children have the freedom to explore social space from every angle of the
imagination. By exploring their physical environments freely with
the body, and their social environments freely with the mind, children use
the free play of imagination to become *oriented from the inside out*. This
body-based metaphorical foundation equips us to navigate paths later
through life based on the inner counsel of intuition as it aligns with outer
flows of information. During psychotherapy, opportunities to build new

structure through play often follow rupture and repair. As therapists, we may rely too much on formulaic or evidence-based approaches, which can snuff out spontaneity and rob us of opportunities to nurture imagination and self-expression in a safe, open-ended playground.

Chapter 8 presents clinical intuition as a major vehicle for the development and expression of wisdom. Wisdom involves the pragmatics of a life well lived, including expertise that is practical, useful, and individually tailored. The domain of wisdom overlaps substantially with core endeavors of psychotherapy: how to assign meaning to ongoing experience, find direction in life, and orchestrate a developmental path toward excellence. Despite popular stereotypes, many therapists have sound vision, great intelligence, and insightful comments, although not all therapists are wise. Within psychotherapy, wisdom goes beyond excellent care of others to include excellent care of self. It is important that as therapists we "walk the talk," by embodying our own ideals, values, and visions. A final clinical case illustrates wisdom in action.

CHAPTER 1

Flashes, Hunches, and Gut Feelings

Intuition is like a slow motion machine that captures data instantaneously and hits you like a ton of bricks.
—Abella Arthur

If the single man plant himself indomitably on his instincts, and there abide, the huge world will come round to him.
—Ralph Waldo Emerson

WHEN YOU ARE WRITING A book on any topic, a natural place to start is to see what already exists. Much to my amazement, I found only one other book about clinical intuition that is specific to the practice of psychotherapy (Charles, 2005), although several authors have touched on the topic (e.g., Bohart, 1999; Myers, 2002; Rosenblatt & Thickstun, 1994; Welling, 2005). There are also plenty of books about the value of intuition to everyday life (e.g., Bastick, 2003; Hogarth, 2001; Rosanoff, 1991; Thibodeau, 2005; Vaughan, 1979), including accuracies and biases of split-second decision-making, sometimes called "thin slicing" (e.g., Claxton, 1997; Gladwell, 2005). I found this absence of relevant material extraordinary. The more I thought about it, the more extraordinary it seemed. Rachel Charles, the author of the other book on this subject, also marveled at the paucity of research. Surprise deepened into disbelief as I crystallized the stance of this book: No matter what their orientation, no matter what their modality, all clinicians tend to use clinical intuition as a nonspecific mode of perception and response during the *actual practice* of psychotherapy.

This book coheres around the following three assumptions:

- Clinical intuition fills the gap between theory and practice during moment-to-moment clinical perception and action;
- Clinical intuition involves attuned detection and response to interpersonal patterns within a healing relationship; and
- Clinical intuition is necessary for deep change within psychotherapy.

The remainder of this chapter lays out these themes broadly.

THE GAP BETWEEN CLINICAL
THEORY AND PRACTICE

Throughout our careers, we clinicians accumulate a body of knowledge. We take continuing education courses to renew clinical licenses and keep up with the latest research. We read and embrace theory to choose clinical orientations and adopt developmental perspectives that inform our concept of psychopathology and health. (As an example, attachment, regulation, and evolutionary theories serve as the foundation for this book.) We accumulate a set of practical facts and principles relevant to the nuts and bolts of practice: ethical standards, how to keep records, the importance of starting and stopping on time, what it means to keep boundaries, and so forth. Finally, we amass ongoing case narratives in the form of session notes, insurance documents, clinical presentations, journal articles, supervision tales, plus running mental dialogues during and between sessions.

Abstract, practical, and case-specific clinical theory is all part of the explicit domain occupied by the conscious, verbal workings of the left hemisphere of the brain. Using theory for guidance during clinical work involves "top-down" processing. When we process from the top down, we start with an idea, schema, or expectation that organizes overall perception and subsequent action. The well-worn psychoanalytic joke "Sometimes a cigar is just a cigar" (see Figure 1.1) hints at one danger of top-down processing when working with patients—projection. If we begin with a fixed assumption that all utterances contain surface material that masks repressed, forbidden sexual content, then a cigar is never a cigar to a therapist, but it always symbolizes a penis.

When we process clinical material in "top-down" fashion, abstract concepts represent a "higher" level than concrete details supplied by minute-to-minute emotional and sensory data. During top-down processing, we do not look with open minds; we look instead to confirm our starting assumptions and presumptions in reductionist fashion. I might approach clinical work with a fixed idea about the meaning of certain symptoms. Perhaps every time I encounter the following cluster within a patient—hypervigilance toward others, enhanced startle reactions, intense pre-

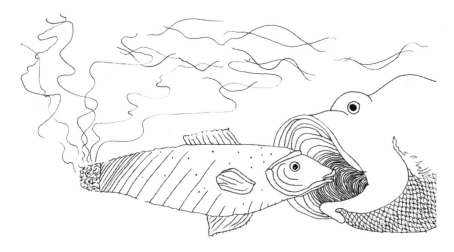

Sometimes a cigar is just a cigar...

Figure 1.1. This drawing provides a triple entendre in the form of a metaphor. Can you identify all three meanings? The foundation is the work of Magritte, who painted a fish with a smoking tail in "L' Exception." The title mocks reductive Freudian symbolism, where long pointy objects, such as cigars, were conceived always to symbolize penises. Finally a cigar is not always a cigar, if it refers to the Bill Clinton/Monica Lewinsky scandal. (Courtesy of the author)

occupation with whatever could go wrong—I assume that somewhere in the past history of my patient's life there exists a traumatic life event. Next I am likely to "look for" the source of trauma in my patient by probing for a specific event. If I fail to find what I am looking for, I may persist in my conviction anyway. I might assume my patient has repressed a troubling memory. While this theory is reasonable, it precludes other possibilities just as likely, if not more. Rather than indicating one big trauma, these same symptoms often arise out of relational trauma (Schore, 2001) borne of a myriad of tiny emotional misattunements, often extending back to early infancy. Another alternative is that these symptoms indicate second-generation posttraumatic stress inherited through social channels.

A classic study by Bugelski and Alampay (1961) revealed the power of feed-forward systems where higher-level information shapes lower levels, not just to influence our ideas, but also the very perception of what we see. Subjects were initially exposed to slides of one of two types of line drawings. Half were exposed to animals, and half to faces. Those who saw animals were much more likely to perceive a rat in the ambiguous drawing in Figure 1.2; those who saw faces tended to perceive a man wearing glasses instead.

CLEARING THE SLATE

The power of preexisting concepts to bias subsequent experience prompted Wilfred Bion, a British psychoanalyst, to emphasize the importance of *not-knowing* as the necessary state of mind during psychotherapy (Bion, 1967). By suggesting that we "set aside all memory and desire" before each session, Bion recommended we clear out ideas derived from the past, along with hopes and projections that reach toward the future. By pointing toward a present-centered form of awareness, Bion highlighted the importance of intuition, as described by the psychoanalyst Steven Ellman:

> The psychoanalyst should aim at achieving a state of mind so that at every session he feels he has not seen the patient before" ([Bion, 1967], p. 18). Therefore, the analyst's "understanding" of what is going on regarding the

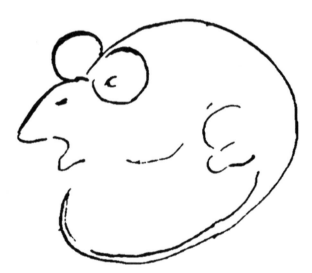

Figure 1.2. What was your first impression—is it a mouse or a man wearing glasses? How long did it take before you were able to switch your perceptual set and see the other figure? The switch, governed by the implicit level, is not entirely subject to willpower, but it instead seems to have a mind of its own. (Original line drawing from Bugelski & Alampay, 1961)

transference, projective identification, thinking, or attacks of linking will only cohere out of the evolution of a selected fact that emerges from experience. As he [Bion] says, "The only point of importance in any session is the unknown. Nothing must be allowed to distract from *intuiting* that (*ibid.*, p. 17)." (2010, pp. 535–536)

When we are sitting before a real person in a real moment, in order to be effective and therapeutic, we need to adopt an open, inquisitive frame of mind. By grounding ourselves in inner sensory, emotional, and imaginal faculties, we can tap into a receptive mode of consciousness. This prepares the mind, brain, and body for the possibility of deep connections with patients that coexist with deep connections with ourselves. Moltu, Binder, and Nielsen described a research study by Geller and Greenberg that offered a model for the ideal therapeutic stance:

> They found that "therapeutic presence involves a careful balancing of contact with the therapist's own experience and contact with the client's experience" (p. 83), and argue that presence involves a *being with* rather than a *doing to* mode of interaction. Our participants' understanding of helpful subjective presence supports these conclusions from Geller and Greenberg (2002), emphasizing the dual qualities of staying open for what comes up in the experiential world and at the same time recognizing the otherness of the patient. (2010, p. 317)

In order to *be with* our patients rather than to *do to* and manipulate them according to preordained experience, we must stay close to ongoing subjective experience (see Figure 1.3). By necessity and design, this opens up a gap between theory and practice within psychotherapy. With regard to the actual clinical hour, no matter how many books we read, no matter how much we think about our cases or how complete our notes may be, there is a limit to where theory can take us with patients. Each of us faces the inevitable chasm between theory and practice that cannot be bridged by ideas alone. In fact, to cling to idea-driven strategies can actually interfere with the clinical process, rendering our responses rote, mechanical, or insensitive to nuance and detail.

IMPLICIT PROCESSES

Clinical intuition contrasts with conscious deliberation in that it is a *bottom-up* mode of processing information that begins with primary sensory, emotional, and other body-based experience as the foundation for organizing immediate response and higher-order perception. As opposed to explicit learning and memory tapped into by conscious thought and theory, clinical intuition taps into implicit processes in the body and brain.

The implicit realm, the subject of Chapter 2, involves a nonconscious form of embodied learning and memory derived from sensorimotor and

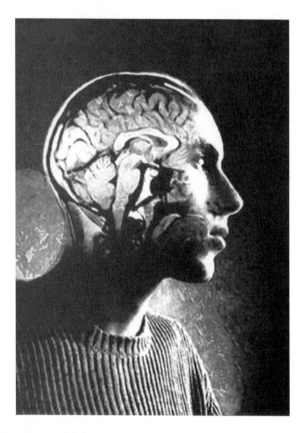

Figure 1.3. It would be wonderful if our patients were completely transparent and we could see inside their heads. Or would it? In reality this sort of merger fantasy puts unrealistic pressure on therapists to know what cannot be known. What is more, we must be careful of what we wish for. If we could read one another's minds, we would not need verbal communication at all. (Public domain: "Inside My Head" by Andrew Mason)

affective experiences. The implicit realm includes procedural memory, which consists of motor sequences such as skipping, leaping, or taking a drink of water. This realm also includes emotional memory that derives from relational sequences beginning within the first hour of the first day of postnatal life. Implicit processes rely on fast-acting subcortical events that permit learning that is both automatic and effort-free within the context of ongoing experience (see Figure 1.4). Developmentally, this allows the infant to internalize sequences of self-in-relation-to-other plus other-in-relation-to-self. By internalizing sequences rather than states, the infant

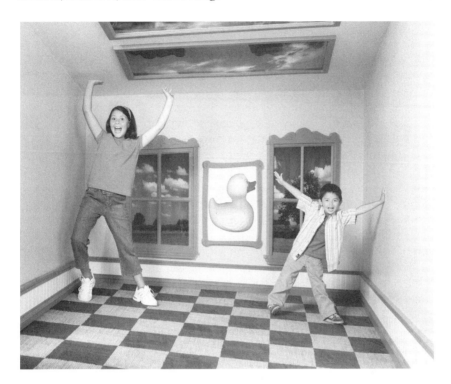

Figure 1.4. Because the implicit realm, including procedural memory, develops long before the explicit realm, children learn most effectively when they participate with their whole bodies. This is what makes exploratory spaces such as the Ames Room so powerful. The Ames Room creates an optical illusion. While it appears to be an ordinary cube from the front, its true trapezoidal shape makes the person on the left appear to be a giant, while the person on the right seems to be a midget. This becomes an embodied lesson about the importance of perspective, something we therapists know much about. (Ames Room, Courtesy of the Strong Museum)

is poised to anticipate what is coming next based on what has come before. Attachment security builds largely through the familiarity of positive expectations confirmed.

Within psychotherapy, implicit processes allow us to assess and respond to patients automatically, without thought. When in a flow, our bodies seem to evaluate what is going on and formulate what to say (or not say) without need for conscious intervention. I have especially noticed that with seasoned practitioners, it becomes common to make an intervention first and *then* stop and think, "Wow! I was right on target.

Where did *that* come from? I didn't know I knew that!" For me, such moments are especially common during clinical supervision, when I find myself espousing broad principles I had not recognized before. One example is "Most of the therapeutic action happens at the edges—at the boundaries between people and transitions between states and events." Another example is "During the first session with patients, try to 'name and reign in.' That is, anticipate patient defenses, especially as based on past therapy experiences. This provides the opportunity to reign in enactments from the start."

During psychotherapy, implicit processes capitalize on brain plasticity, because therapists and patients alike internalize interactive sequences. Hopefully, the reactivity of early negative and traumatic sequences is counteracted with the responsiveness of more positive, growth-promoting ones. Moment-to-moment intuition requires a shuttling back and forth of attention, between self and other, inner and outer worlds, past and present, present and future. As we shift attention between different modes, scales, contents, and processes during the psychotherapy, clinicians continually make distinctions between what arises from within and what arises from outside the self. In order to make such distinctions, we must ground ourselves in embodied self-awareness.

EMBODIED AWARENESS

"Embodied awareness" is the phrase that Alan Fogel (2009) used to highlight the body-based stream of self-awareness, as it contrasts with a second, more thought-based stream he called "conceptual self-awareness." Whereas conceptual self-awareness is frozen in time and slow to change, embodied self-awareness is ever in flux, shifting rapidly in response to moment-to-moment relational dynamics. This never-ending dance of defining and re-defining inner and outer boundaries requires that therapists pay close attention to body signals. First we look inward, using what Damasio (1996, 1999) called *somatic markers*, and then we look outward to *read* the faces and bodies of our patients. Through the right hemisphere we tune in to the music of our own emotions and minds, and then we re-tune in order to hear the melody under the words of our patients. Through intuitive processing within the implicit realm, we engage in a nonstop, dynamic dance of dual awareness, continually making tiny shifts and micro-adjustments in attention and response on the basis of embodied awareness.

Over the course of evolution, the continual expansion of both right and left cerebral cortices has lent ever greater complexity and flexibility to animal responses. But the right hemisphere is best at retaining the overview necessary for the kind of dual attention we use as psychotherapists. In particular, it is the job of the orbitofrontal lobes to monitor both internal and external environments, as well as to attend to shifts of attention in the process (Barbas, 2007). Whereas the left hemisphere processes the right side of space only, the right processes both sides (see Figure 1.5; McGilchrist, 2009). The left cerebral hemisphere zooms in on one thing at a time. By operating in serial fashion, the left attends well to parts of experience, reducing the full complexity of a scene in order to lock down the details. In this way, the left hemisphere *looks for* things and readily sacrifices the forest for the trees along its deductive path. That is why it represents the essence of a top-down approach.

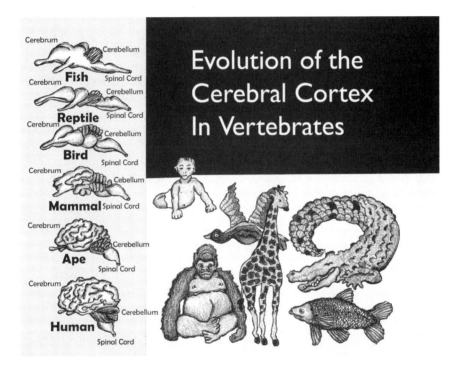

Figure 1.5. This drawing depicts the evolution of the cerebral cortex in vertebrates. There was an evolutionary trend from a smooth texture of the cerebral hemispheres, or cerebrum, to ever more complex folds allowing for a greater and greater amount of surface area to be packed into a small space inside the skull. Within mammals, the two hemispheres became more and more specialized, or lateralized, through evolution. While scientists used to think that different hemispheres specialize according to what task is being performed, it appears more likely that both sides are capable of carrying out all tasks. Instead, the two hemispheres enjoy different perspectives on the world. (Courtesy of the author.)

By contrast the holistic perspective of the right hemisphere places it in a better position *to look at* things in an open fashion. This allows clinicians to pay attention to what becomes emotionally salient from moment to moment based on the immediate feedback of ongoing, embodied experience. Along with tiny fluctuations in attention during micro-moments, the right hemisphere also drives the higher-order, large-scale inductive path by which insight puts together multisensory pieces of information (McCrea, 2010).

Here is a clinical example of how the right hemisphere shifts our clinical attention. A patient is telling me about a phone call to his mother. Suddenly my attention gets drawn to the man's wildly tapping leg. I feel compelled to interrupt his narrative to switch our collective focus to what his body communicates. We link the man's leg gestures to intense anger expressed toward his mother in a previous session. Although he would have liked to kick his mother then, anger is currently missing from the patient's awareness and narrative. Consciously he may deny that he is upset. He may make all sorts of excuses for his mother's insensitivity at this point in time, when perhaps guilt has set in. Yet, unconsciously, anger still lurks in the patient's body in the form of a violently vibrating leg. It is the right hemisphere that notices the unexpressed emotion and orchestrates these switches in attention. It is the right hemisphere that combines and unifies these fragments of ongoing experience, based on the full context of what is most emotionally salient.

INTUITION IN THE RIGHT BRAIN

Among researchers who locate intuition as a right-brain mode, Iain McGilchrist, a British psychiatrist, emphasized the relative independence of the two hemispheres. The corpus callosum is the wide flat bundle of nerve fibers located between the two cerebral hemispheres, and it consists of 200–250 million contralateral axonal projections (see Figure 1.6). Most of its fibers are excitatory physiologically, and this large mass of white body in the brain certainly facilitates interhemispheric communication by coordinating corresponding sides of the body and structures in the brain.

Yet because the brain is fundamentally nonlinear (Glanz, 1997; Kitzbichler, Smith, Christensen, & Bullmore, 2009), and tiny differences sometimes mobilize a huge impact, the corpus callosum simultaneously serves the broad function of inhibiting the perspective of one hemisphere in order to bring to the fore the other. McGilchrist asserted that this inhibitory role affects not just *how we look* at things, but the very world that we bring into being.

McGilchrist's book *The Master and His Emissary: The Divided Brain and the Making of the Western World* drew its name from a Nietzsche story about a master and his emissary. The master is so successful at rul-

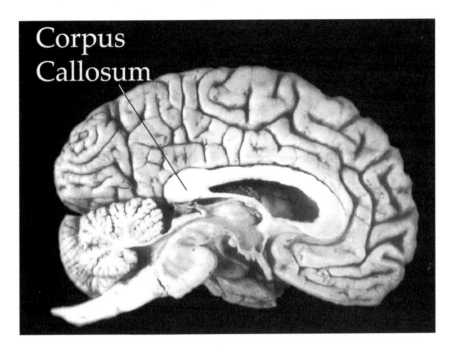

Figure 1.6. The corpus callosum in a mid-sagital cut of the brain. Although it is not apparent in this image, the two hemispheres are not perfectly symmetrical. Instead, the right side has a slight bulge in front, while the left side has a slight bulge in back. These bulges correspond to important differences in specialization. Whereas the right front specializes in executive functions, the back left specializes in language-related functions.

ing the land that his territory grows and grows until it gets so big that the master becomes removed from the everyday affairs of the people. This enables the emissary to feel erroneously that it is he and not his master in charge of the land as a whole. McGilchrist likened this story to relations between the left and right cerebral hemispheres. Because the left holds explicit knowledge in consciousness, far removed from the supportive implicit underpinnings of the fundamentally nonconscious operations of the right side, it erroneously conceives of itself in charge of the whole, while losing sight of the less visible, body-based, integrative functions of the right. Einstein came up with a similar metaphor: "Intuition is a sacred gift. Rationality its faithful servant. We have created a society that honors the servant and has forgotten the gift."

Within psychotherapy, we continually shuttle back and forth between the intuitive mode of the right hemisphere and the deliberative mode of the left one. Here, too, it is the intuitive right side that integrates the whole. When the left hemisphere is dominant, so is its primary motive—power (Kuhl & Kazén, 2008). Power is facilitated by instrumental, mono-semantic (single-focus) processing of the left hemisphere. During social interactions, this approach *reduces* appraisals of people to the single aspect most fitting with one's purposes. Within the clinical setting, left-brain approaches easily evoke the feeling of "being done to." As Kuhl and Kazén put it, "Close relationships can even be disturbed when one of the interaction partners displays explicit means-end intentionality (e.g., uses the other person to accomplish a goal)" (p. 467).

By contrast to the power motive of the left, the right cerebral hemisphere is characterized by an affiliation motive. The holistic, polysemantic (multiple-focus) processing style of the right hemisphere (Beeman, Friedman, Grafman, Perez, Diamond, & Lindsay, 1994; Rotenberg, 2004) preserves the wholeness of others; it honors their multidimensional nature while retaining the full complexity of the clinical encounter. This facilitates the I-Thou relationship of highest respect, as conceived by the philosopher Martin Buber, in contrast to the I-It relationship of the marketplace.

Clearly there is a place for deliberation, strategy, problem solving, and other modes of conscious, explicit processing during every clinical hour, just as there is a place for invoking a power motive, when we make decisions or even take over on behalf of a patient's welfare, in service of the relationship. But as a general stance, most therapists would probably choose affiliation over power as the primary motive for working with patients. And even here we still get into trouble unconsciously if power motives creep to the fore unwittingly, as when we try to "fix" our patients or change them due to our own discomforts and defensive needs.

Different therapeutic modalities vary in the degree to which these two motives are highlighted. Cognitive-behavioral therapists are more comfortable assuming the power of authority by adopting a more directive stance. By contrast, relationally oriented therapists on the whole are less interested in orchestrating behavior than in harnessing the natural healing and growth afforded by solid attachment within a context of trust. But within all modalities, ultimately both hemispheres have to work together, especially given evidence that the more creativity a complex problem requires, the more both hemispheres come into play for a solution (Jaušovec, 2000). Psychotherapy is one of the most complex endeavors around, and during moment-to-moment clinical work, awareness continually shuttles back and forth between the two modes. In clinical examples throughout this book, especially those that include moment-to-moment dynamics, I highlight the necessity of shuttling back and forth in many directions—between inner versus outer worlds, embodied versus conceptual self-awareness, feeling versus thought, and intuitive versus deliberating modes.

THE THERAPEUTIC ENCOUNTER

When clinical intuition draws on the primary stuff of the eyes, ears, bodily sensations, and emotions to fill the gap between theory and practice, it enters the territory of Daniel Stern's (2004) "now" moments of therapy. Now moments involve the ongoing feel of things as they are processed at a micro-scale of analysis. Through the magnifying lens of the subjective present, nothing stays still. One minute, a patient beams with the joy of self-revelation, only to collapse under a wave of shame triggered by a slight wince detected on the face of the therapist. There is a never-ending kaleidoscope of ever-shifting self-states in patient and therapist alike (see Figure 1.7). These states sometimes blend, collide, synchronize, or repel. Moments of contact come and go amid continually changing contours of perception, motivation, and emotion. Negatively and positively tinged exchanges vary in intensity and arousal levels. In order to give readers the feel for ever-shifting intuitive moments during psychotherapy, in chapters to come, I include snippets of clinical dialogue whenever possible.

Social Patterns—Attuned Perception and Response

Clinical intuition may fill the gap between theory and practice, but with what? While in intuitive mode, what is it that we perceive? We perceive and respond to ever-shifting interpersonal patterns. The function of intuition is to allow in novel information that arises from moment-to-moment shifts in the emotional contours of the therapeutic relationship.

Therefore, the content of intuition is highly idiosyncratic. Indeed, personal differences between therapists, such as the capacity for empathy, may be of greater importance to clinical results than differences based on theoretical orientation. Early outcome research, such as conducted by Hans Strupp (1978), focused on personality differences between therapists. More recent evidence suggests that a robust therapist effect in psychotherapy process and outcome can far exceed differences between therapeutic methods (Dinger, Strack, Leichsenring, Wilmers, & Schauenberg, 2008; Hupert et al., 2001; Lutz, Leon, Martinovich, Lyons, & Stiles, 2007; Wampold, 2010; Wampold & Brown, 2005).

Given findings of greater variation within rather than between different theoretical schools, contemporary studies often seek pan-theoretical factors spread across all orientations. One of these factors is the quality of the therapeutic relationship. Nissen-Lie, Monsen, and Ronnestad (2010) examined the therapist's contribution to the working alliance. Characteristics most predictive of a strong working alliance involved relational skills. Therapists perceived by patients as warm, accepting, engaged, empathic, and responsive appear best able to establish strong working

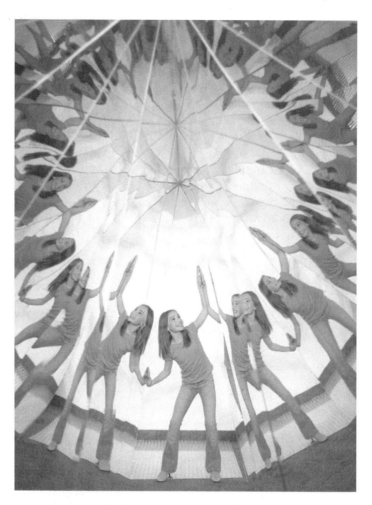

Figure 1.7. A kaleidoscope serves as an excellent visual metaphor for the ever-shifting interpersonal patterns that therapists pick up through clinical intuition. Just like in a kaleidoscope, the old bits of experience get shaken up and recombined in new ways, lending a quality of familiarity along with that of novelty. (Courtesy of the Strong Museum)

alliances. From the neurobiological point of view of underlying structures, warm engagement and empathy include not just a cognitive dimension of understanding but also an emotional dimension. In this way, we go beyond simple knowing to emotional involvement and feeling for what our patients feel (e.g., Lamm, Bateson, & Decety, 2007).

Clinical intuition is a form of social and emotional intelligence (Goleman, 1997) that contributes to a strong working alliance. Through clinical intuition, we detect and respond to relational patterns both within our patients and within ourselves. In order to perceive patterns within a healing context, clinicians need to know, and just as importantly to feel, the minds of others. Sometimes the melding of the minds takes on rather extraordinary dimensions. Recently, a patient of many years, Sabina, shared the following transference dream about me:

> *You were underwater, waving your arms as if holding paintbrushes in both hands you used to create swirling shapes on pieces of paper, one for each hand. As each painting was completed, the papers floated upwards towards the surface. Suddenly among all the papers, the dead body of an adolescent boy also floated upwards. You kissed the back of his neck. The boy's eyes popped open and suddenly he came alive. I woke up. The dream was so scary. The images stayed with me for hours. I couldn't get back to sleep.*

This dream was a concrete illustration of what Kestenberg (1985) called "dead spots" in the infant's subjective experience. Indeed the dream, along with the associations it stirred, wound up "bringing alive" a realm of dissociated emotion connected to previously unrepressed but unprocessed sexual trauma that occurred during Sabina's adolescence. When she first relayed the dream, I could visualize the images clearly—to the point of describing some unspoken details. What is more, I *felt the dream images in my body*. Interestingly, I felt the images not as myself, but as Sabina watching me, as she did in her dream. I believe strong resonances such as these set the foundation for sensitivity during the explorations that followed.

All the theory in the world will not produce effective clinical work if a therapist lacks the capacity for empathy by which we put ourselves into the shoes of others. Through empathy, we intuitively feel our way into the emotional and motivational states of patients. By seeing the world through their eyes, we can better understand the roles and rules of their relationships and how these come into play in the moment-to-moment dynamics of the session (see Figure 1.8).

Empathic Roots

The empathic roots of clinical intuition can be traced back to the mammalian attachment system, where instincts to nurture, love, and bond with others facilitate our understanding of them. Human babies are born with brains and nervous systems that are immature. From the start, babies need attuned responses by which caregivers understand what they are feeling and needing. The prolific work of Allan Schore (e.g., 2003a, 2003b) has been instrumental in illuminating the importance of the first two years of life for laying the right-brain foundations for behavioral, emotional, social, and cognitive development throughout life. This is the time

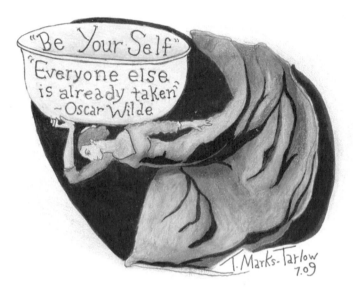

Figure 1.8. Conceptual self-awareness puts experience into conceptual boxes according to preformed categories. In this way, thought and language are both aspects of conceptual awareness that operate by reducing the complexity of experience to simpler forms, which then can be manipulated independent of their original context. As therapists, we draw upon conceptual awareness, for example, to diagnose patients. By contrast, embodied self-awareness always occurs in context and so it is rich in detail that renders each moment unique. As therapists, we use embodied awareness in the throes of clinical intuition by tracking minute-to-minute state fluctuations. With embodied self-awareness as the foundation for conceptual self-awareness, this drawing takes inspiration from the words of Oscar Wilde and the movement of Martha Graham, urging us to relish our uniqueness. (Courtesy of the author)

when internal working models of relationships get established implicitly through the workings of the emotional, relational, intuitive right brain. Schore highlights right-brain to right-brain communication between parent and baby. When parents speak and sing to their babies, it is the nonverbal right-brain to right-brain communication that shapes the contours of the underlying implicit communication.

Through the emotional dimension of empathy, clinicians frequently resonate with emotions expressed. If a patient reports a significant trauma or loss, we tend to feel an attenuated version of his or her pain or terror. We may mirror the contours of our patients' emotions, without reaching their intensity. This way, we can remain emotionally regulated, even if our patients may not be. But empathy extends even further—at times touching on emotions that remain unexpressed. Precisely because clinical intuition operates on implicit levels, we are just as likely to resonate with dissociated emotion as we are to resonate with that which is fully embodied into conscious awareness.

When dissociated emotion hovers and is picked up by therapists, we serve as "tuning forks" (Stone, 2006) in the intersubjective space between the patient and therapist. When this occurs, it is through clinical intuition by which we pick up on these nuances. We journey inward to detect emotion and then try to parcel out the self from the other as best we can. There is even the radical suggestion (Ginot, 2009) that enactments between therapist and patient, by which each is caught in reactive sequences, sometimes represent empathic attunements at the unconscious level of dissociated emotion. When this occurs, we resonate with emotion that may be more wholly the patient's than our own.

Here is a recent example. I had an initial session with a well-dressed, high-functioning doctor. On the surface, little of emotional significance occurred. Much of that first hour, the man conscientiously relayed background information. His affect was neutral but pleasant, and his style methodical and patient. Underneath and inexplicably, I flew into a panic. By the end of the session I was afraid for my very life. I was not afraid *of* the patient; in fact, there was no specific content associated with my state of mind. I simply hit some level of primitive terror connected with basic survival.

My emotional experience felt meaningful but made little intellectual sense, until several sessions later when things clicked into place as I learned a critical piece of his history. As an only child and son of a military family, the man had been left by his parents to fend for himself with peers. This was considered a matter of honor and what it meant to be a man. For several years during elementary school as a boy my patient had been bullied by several older boys who repeatedly stalked him after school. My patient was frequently chased, beat-up, and left feeling *scared for his life*, yet he learned not to turn to anyone for help. He learned how to suppress his fear and pain and to tuck away all signs of vulnerability.

Over time, these defenses had hardened and had reached such extremes that the man repetitively left all relationships as his only means *to reclaim vitality*. As I took in these details, I suddenly understood what had happened to me that first session. As this man prepared to enter into a new, potentially life-altering relationship with me, I was left feeling the terror he held deep down inside his body, but did not yet have the resources to consciously bear/bare. Psychologically, this seemed to be a case of empathy through embodied countertransference. My body served as the tuning fork or resonant chamber for all of the dissociated emotion this man had yet to feel.

GROWTH THROUGH PLAY

One avenue for empathy to develop is through play. When an attuned mother tickles her newborn's toes, she intuitively chooses a moment when he is alert, open for stimulation, and ready to receive and reciprocate the positive emotion of joy. From an attachment perspective, when a mother soothes negative emotion, including repairing a relationship following rupture, she instills a sense of safety and trust that brings the baby back to emotional equilibrium. By reducing arousal and restoring the baby's comfort, the mother has now cleared the deck for the baby's interest in play. A host of developmental literature reveals that *play is the work of childhood*. Play is where novelty thrives, insofar as new cognitive, behavioral, and social skills are most likely to emerge. Vygotsky (1978, 1986) proposed unstructured imaginative play to serve as a "zone of proximal development" where children try out their leading edges of growth. During play, there is freedom to take risks safely, without dire consequences. As later chapters illustrate, novelty can be explored intuitively, within the context of imagination.

Following in the footsteps of the British psychoanalyst Donald Winnicott (1971) and, more recently, the Australian psychoanalyst Russell Meares (2005), I have introduced a play model of clinical intuition and structure building within psychotherapy. Whereas negative emotions are primarily constrictive and oriented toward defense and self-protection (Frederickson, 1998, 2001) positive emotions are expansive while building resources. Interest, curiosity, passion, and joy are all cultivated through play, as perspective taking is learned and timing is mastered relationally. The capacity to incorporate novelty without defense is a hallmark of mental health, as well as of play. Early play involves not only developing skills necessary for later adulthood, but also interpersonal skills related to emotional development, risk taking, and the capacity to tolerate the kinds of emotional intensity associated with learning new things and recovering after losses.

The urge to play is a key aspect of clinical intuition, partly because it runs so deep within the instinctive urges of most species of mammals, especially those that live in groups. Play may be less likely to characterize short-term, symptom-focused therapy, but it is more important when transitioning to long-term, open-ended psychotherapy. Especially once people get beyond a survival orientation toward the work, heightened curiosity plus a playful spirit may be required to sustain interest in further growth. Interestingly, the play instinct in mammals (as shown in Figure 1.9) even includes a rupture-and-repair sequence (Bekoff & Pierce, 2009) that mirrors moment-to-moment explorations and risk taking within our offices.

There is continuity between early games of infancy and childhood and later forms they take when reappearing within clinical exchanges. Hide-and-seek is the prototypical game of psychotherapy, as explored in

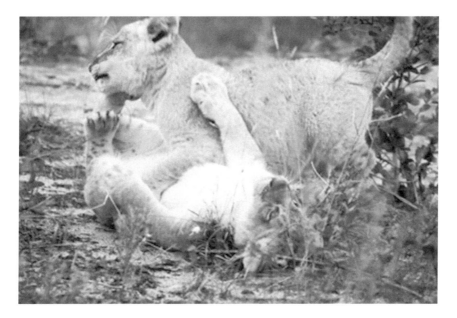

Figure 1.9. Two lion cubs at play. (Courtesy of Jimmy Wales)

Chapter 4. Patients typically seek help because they want to be seen and known, yet they often hide from therapists and themselves, out of fear and shame. Within the hide-and-seek of psychotherapy, different implicit rules emerge with each patient-therapist pair. Sometimes the therapist must chase the patient, through offers of insight, interpretations, suggestions, and so on, while the patient runs away to hide in the safety of isolation. At other times, the patient and therapist join together at conscious levels of cooperation, collaboratively seeking more unconscious levels of self. Within psychotherapy, games like this are often far from fun, yet they remain a cornerstone of clinical interchanges, including attempts to shed outdated defenses.

Apart from games with rules, therapists regularly use the play of intuition to help patients heal and become more oriented within intersubjective space. Even amid painful emotions and heartbreaking experiences, we often move out of the joy of exploration and self-discovery, as well as fascination and interest afforded by discovering and addressing intrapsychic and interpersonal patterns. As therapists, these positive motives, even amid negative emotion, help keep us refreshed and vital and protected against therapist burnout. Just as laughter and humor are central to children's play, so, too, laughter and humor are important to any therapist's bag of tricks (see Figure 1.10). Humor and laughter relate to safety,

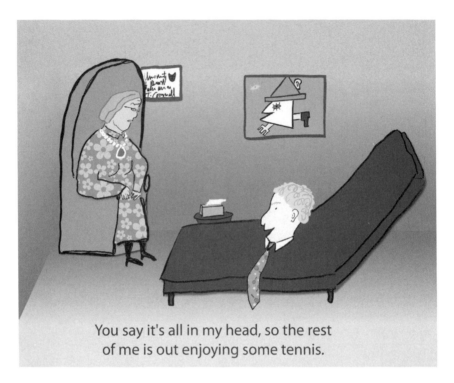

You say it's all in my head, so the rest
of me is out enjoying some tennis.

Figure 1.10. Victor Yalom, the creator of this cartoon, is a clinical psychologist based in San Francisco who likes to play with serious subjects within psychotherapy through the use of humor. Few therapists would assert that what a patient expresses is "all in his head." This amounts to telling someone he is "crazy." In fact, by emphasizing the subcortical, somatic elements of embodied experience at the basis of clinical intuition, this book could go to the opposite extreme to assert "it's all in your body." (© 2011 Victor Yalom/Psychotherapy.net)

spontaneity, surprise, and creativity, which are all part of the territory of intuition. Laughter can increase bonding and a sense of a common universe, along with providing an opportunity for perspective sharing. Additionally, laughter often signals the release of trauma on the verge of building a new internal structure.

CLINICAL INTUITION AS THE ROYAL ROAD TO CHANGE

From a nonlinear perspective, psychotherapy is a two-way street. We therapists often become enriched and grow alongside our patients (Marks-

Tarlow, 2008a). One implication of such circular feedback loops and causality is that the intuitive mode is not just important to therapists. Intuition is just as critical to the healing of patients. Much like the implicit realm of body-based awareness and response is central for inner guidance within therapists, so, too, does this same mode facilitate self-trust and free expression within patients. In fact, the ability to bypass explicit levels in order to tap into implicit processes often is the missing piece for patients.

Many patients enter psychotherapy with a consciously formulated understanding of what is wrong; they may even know what they need to do about it. Consider an overweight person who already knows she needs to lose weight. She has the best of intentions and makes plans. Yet she remains unable to embody her knowledge fully in order to live it. What is an ordinary divide between explicit and implicit realms becomes especially deep if primary emotion is suppressed or dissociated from awareness, in which case nonconscious aspects tend to run the body's show. This gap easily triggers shame in the overweight person who knows what she has to do, but is unable to execute what otherwise appears so simple. People with a good grasp of explicit but not implicit realms can feel particularly demoralized and self-blaming.

To engage clinical intuition in service of our patients learning how to engage their own intuitive mode is often the cornerstone to therapeutic progress. When patients move according to their own inner vision and counsel, they can orient themselves according to holistic faculties afforded by the right brain. By processing and producing more novelty, patients use more of their inner resources to become grounded and more expansive. They are in a better position to shed constricting defenses, face risks, and to process novelty and even seek it out. When embedded within the embodied, relational, emotional faculties of the right brain, imagination becomes a portal into healing as well as into new states of reality rather than as a haven for fantasy or an escape. This is the subject of Chapter 6.

CHANGE WITHOUT INSIGHT

Although insight is definitely an aspect of clinical intuition, I concord with others, such as Lyons-Ruth (1998) and Schore (2011), who believe insight is not always necessary for therapeutic change. When working intuitively with patients, it is possible to affect change without or well before insight. Certainly this holds true for our youngest child patients whose symbolic capacities may not even have developed yet. The possibility for change without insight also holds for many adult patients with the greatest amount of suffering, trauma, dissociation, and emotional dysregulation. Precisely because empathic skills derive from parental instincts that exist in all mammals, they do not depend on words or thought for implementation. The affective foundation for empathy originates at subcortical levels in the brain and the autonomic nervous system.

As a rule of thumb, the more severe the symptoms, the greater the importance of engaging patients in body-to-body fashion, where the primary dynamics involve nonconscious flows of emotion and arousal. In order to reach deep levels where traumatic images and expectations are stored in images, sounds, and other body experiences within implicit processes, empathic resonance must occur at subcortical levels where emotions, motivations, and social expectations originate. This is the basis for body-based treatments of trauma, such as sensorimotor therapy (see Ogden, Minton, & Pain, 2006).

Classical psychoanalysis, as conceived by Freud, began with the assumption that change requires making the unconscious conscious through well-timed interpretations. Over the century since Freud lived, this assumption has been challenged again and again, especially by contemporary relational psychoanalysts who argue for the importance of implicit over explicit processes. Christopher Bollas (1987) tackled early preverbal knowledge by writing about "the unthought known." A case described by Arizmendi (2008) in the chapter to come illustrates the importance of nonverbal exchanges that can lead to change in the absence of insight. Many argue that premature interpretation is a frequent source of ruptures in psychotherapy. This holds especially true for people whose relational trauma began in the crib, however subtly, through tiny emotional misses, intrusions, or lack of reparations, all preceding conscious thought. The humanistic orientation of Gestalt therapy, with its emphasis on direct experience, contact, and experimentation in the moment-to-moment context, was not concerned with insight. But this school of therapy historically was not concerned much with theory either, arising in rebellion from the constrictions and authoritative stance of classical psychoanalysis.

When insight does emerge during clinical work, it tends to do so as a by-product, or derivative, of moment-to-moment immersion that is guided by the subcortical processes of clinical intuition. By understanding that clinical intuition involves *bottom-up* processes, we now have neurobiological tools to model its centrality to change. Whether in the form of images, sounds, metaphors, abstract pattern perception, and sometimes even words, clinical insight often arises independent of conscious thought. This is because the highest levels of symbolism and creativity occur in the right and not left cerebral hemisphere (McGilchrist, 2009; Schore, 2011).

WRAP-UP

This introductory chapter introduced three ways of understanding clinical intuition. First, intuition fills the gap between therapy and practice. By guiding our moment-to-moment perception of patients as focused through the lens of the self, this cleans the slate of top-down preconceptions. We then begin anew, in line with bottom-up, raw data as drawn from embodied experience. As a right-brain mode of information processing, intuition coordinates our switches in attention, our switches between hemispheres, as well as the clinical art of timing. Second, clinical intuition involves the capacity to perceive, process, and respond to social patterns. Through emotional circuits we share with other mammals, the instincts to bond with, nurture, and care for others lend us empathic tools to feel and think our way into the minds of our patients. In this way, clinical intuition is continuous with parental instincts as shared by all social mammals. Finally, clinical intuition is an inner faculty necessary for therapeutic change both in therapists and patients alike. True change requires openness to novelty. This is the bailiwick of the right (and not the left) hemisphere. Transformation during psychotherapy harnesses imagination and creativity. Unless we can conceive of a future that differs from the past, we cannot live one out.

With this whole in mind, chapters to follow expand on these themes, with the goal being to flesh out details, often through extended clinical cases.

CHAPTER 2

Implicit Processes

The power of intuitive understanding will protect you from harm until the end of your days.
—Lao-Tzu

The smallest flower is a thought, a life answering to some feature of the Great Whole, of whom they have a persistent intuition.
—Honoré de Balzac

TO BE IN THE FLOW (Csikszentmihalyi, 1990) of intuition during clinical work is to enter a state of full immersion akin to deep meditation. Regardless of the content of the session, all focus is on *this* relationship in *this* moment in *this* room with *this* person. The flow of clinical intuition also resembles intense engagement during the creative process. Indeed, Csikszentmihalyi (1996) extended the concept of flow to the psychology of discovery and invention. Wherever intuition is at play there is novelty, either in perception or production.

When both the therapist and patient are caught up in a flow, the dynamics can feel like a wave. Moments of contact may come and go but there is an overall sense of momentum. Time can disappear for much of the clinical hour only to burst into awareness near the end, as if cued by an inner alarm clock. A session that carves a well-formed wave is not unlike a drama whose plot crescendos about three-quarters of the way in and winds down for the denouement. Patients instinctively attend to the temporal frame, perhaps due to their reluctance to leave the office in high states of arousal. Yet failure to contain intense affect within the confines of the clinical hour is inevitable at some point during most treatments. These dysregulated periods may themselves represent the crescendo of an even larger wave that extends across the entire course of treatment.

Just as artists have days of deep focus and other days where nothing comes, no clinician remains permanently in a state of flow. Some sessions feel jerky and sputtering. Patients sometimes enter the office feeling recalcitrant, withdrawn, or defended. Power struggles can ensue over who will talk first or who will keep things going. Sometimes the air is filled with tension. An intensely depressed patient may sap a therapist of vitality. Therapists may enter the office preoccupied. Many things can block the intuitive mode of flow. Whether smooth or filled with turbulence the *feel* of a session belongs to the *implicit* realm of psychotherapy.

As talk therapists, we traditionally emphasize the *explicit* level, which includes verbal conscious productions like thoughts, words, and narratives. By attending to the content of communications and analyzing the meaning of words, many forms of psychotherapy target the explicit level. In classical psychoanalysis, for example, patient insight is the point, and analysts deliver well-timed interpretations designed to "make the unconscious conscious." Cognitive-behavioral therapists court the explicit realm by addressing how negative and dysfunctional thoughts drive emotion and behavior. Narrative therapists within the postmodern tradition deconstruct patient narratives, or explicit stories about their lives, in order to reconstruct more adaptive ones. Counseling psychologists and social workers focus on the explicit level by discussing life problems in order to seek and implement solutions.

In contrast to these trends is the growing recognition of the importance of the *implicit* realm (Bucci, 2011; Cortina & Liotti, 2007; Fosshage, 2011; Mancia, 2006; Marks-Tarlow, 2011; Ruth-Lyons, 1998; Schore, 2010, 2011). This especially holds for schools of thought that place the quality of patient-therapist interactions at the center of healing and growth. The Boston Change Process Study Group and New York Relational School are two examples. Spearheaded by the developmental perspective of infant researchers like Daniel Stern, Beatrice Beebe, and Ed Tronick, the self is conceived to develop, thrive, or falter through internalizing implicit relational interactions with caregivers. Not just during childhood, but also throughout the life span, meaning is conveyed in the form of nonverbal information that is sent and picked up by the body. Tone, pitch, pace, and volume of voice; facial expressions; and body gestures are all paralinguistic cues that help children and adults alike to keep running tabs on the feelings, motivations, intentions, fantasies, and expectations of others.

Researchers estimate that 60% of what transpires between people occurs nonverbally through nonverbal, implicit channels (Burgoon, 1985). According to Schore (2011), along with *implicit cognition* (unconscious processing of exteroceptive information from the outer world and interoceptive information from the inner world), implicit processes also include *implicit affect* (emotion registered nonconsciously by the body, which may or may not reach consciousness), *implicit self-regulation* (internal regulation of arousal, affect intensity, and behavioral impulse) and *implicit communication* (facial expressions, postures, and body gestures that communicate underlying emotion and motivation).

In this chapter, I discuss the origins of clinical intuition within the implicit realm. During psychotherapy, intuitive, implicit processes are orchestrating the music of therapy (affective expression through tone, cadence, and rhythm of speech) while choreographing its dance (inclination to gesticulate, shift positions, mirror poses, counteract postures, express emotion facially). Especially when carried by flow states, inspired by imagination or basking in insight, implicit processes can produce the content of responses as well.

Before I present research on implicit memory and implicit learning as it relates to clinical intuition, I will introduce the clinical story of Gus, a case revisited several times in chapters to come, including the final one on wisdom. At this point in the book I intend to give readers a feel for how implicit processes contrast with explicit ones, how important implicit processes are from the onset of psychotherapy, and how we clinicians automatically enfold implicit relational knowledge into our responses. In the dialogue that follows, which occurred during the initial telephone contact, I immediately picked up on and responded to Gus's implicit rather than explicit agenda. If I had not done so, the outcome might have proved disastrous.

DUAL/DUELING REALMS

"Thanks for returning my call. I'm looking for psychotherapy. I will be blunt about my problem and what I'm looking for. Every time I make love with my wife, I experience myself as a woman. Although my wife has no idea that this is going on I'm afraid of losing her. I'm scared that unless I rid myself of this behavior I'll lose my marriage. Can you help me?"

Immediately I felt myself recoil inside, because within Gus's request, I sensed violence he wished to perpetrate on an unwanted aspect of himself. Intuitively and from the start, I experienced this man as asking for something he did not need. I replied, "I seriously doubt that it's possible to rid yourself of this kind of experience. To be honest even if you could, I am not sure it would be a good idea to try."

"What direction would you go instead? How could you help me?"

"I can help you to understand the meaning of your experience" was my response.

"But I'm not interested in insight," shot back Gus. "I just want to change my behavior."

"This isn't just some bad habit you've developed," I protested. "Your experience is a vital part of who you are."

Gus thought for a second and then concluded, "Well, let's set up an initial appointment and see what happens."

When I opened my door for the first session, I found a polite, respectful, attentive, open, and thoughtful 62-year-old man. I liked Gus immediately. He carefully provided background to his problem. Gus was in his second marriage of 15 years with a wife who was 21 years younger. Gus's experience of feeling like a woman first developed around age 36, shortly after his first marriage of 15 years dissolved. I asked him about past psychotherapy. This is one of the few routine questions I have during a first session. The information helps me to identify strengths, pitfalls, and potential impasses quickly. Gus replied that just before contacting me he had tried some psychotherapy for his condition.

"How did it go?" I inquired.

"Not very helpful. The woman showed me to the door within 20 minutes. She diagnosed me with gender identity disorder and then referred me to a gender disorder clinic. The diagnosis didn't feel right—seemed too simplistic. I did some research online. Too much doesn't fit. I have no interest in changing my gender or my body. I like being a man. I'm happy in my relationship with my wife. What do *you* think my diagnosis is?"

When Gus asked me this, I immediately felt resistance inside my jaw, my teeth clenching tightly. "You ask me to diagnose you, but I doubt that would help you now. You just told me the issue of diagnosis was why you left your previous therapy. Besides I have the feeling you aren't going to fit nicely into some standard diagnostic pigeonhole anyway. Even if I wanted to diagnose you—which by the way *does* interest me—it will take me time to do so with any confidence."

As it turned out, not only did Gus's diagnosis take a long time to make, but because his symptoms morphed right along with the treatment, it made no sense to consider diagnosis apart from the relational dynamics of treatment. Initially Gus's experience of himself as a woman began as a habit during masturbation. So, at first we talked about Gus's symptom in terms of something he *did*, a *behavior* he voluntarily initiated. Then as therapy progressed, Gus's habit began to amplify and increase in frequency and so appeared more like a sexual *fetish*. When Gus's experience expanded beyond masturbation, his symptom next appeared more like a method of reducing stress broadly and we began talking about his experience of himself as a woman as a *fantasy*. Then Gus's contact with his female side became more autonomous, taking on a life of its own. At times the switch might envelop Gus's entire body, at other times just a single finger. It was at this point that we came to understand these states of mind/body/brain to involve Gus's *dissociation* from integral aspects of his *being*, arising out of relational trauma.

I return to Gus's case frequently in this book to highlight different aspects and phases of treatment. But here my intention is to underscore the dynamic and fluid nature of Gus's presenting complaint. I previously wrote about Gus (Marks-Tarlow, 2011) in a paper for *Psychoanalytic Dialogues* that applied principles from nonlinear science to the practice of psychoanalysis. I chose this case because of the complex relationship between diagnosis and treatment that flies in the face of the Western medical model. One reason that clinical intuition is so vital to psychotherapy is precisely because of this complex relationship.

Psychoanalysis arose over a century ago in Europe within a mechanistic model that is both linear and reductionistic. Each step—diagnosis, prescription, treatment, and follow-up—derives logically from the previous one. Information is gathered through careful observation, a medical history, and tests aimed at differential diagnosis. Each step attempts to minimize medical uncertainty. Yet with Gus this was all turned around. Diagnosis did not precede treatment in a predictable, stepwise progression. A course of treatment was not implied reductionistically by his diagnosis. The rush toward certainty was part of the problem and not the solution. Gus needed help resisting his own intellectual curiosity in order to reside in the ambiguity rather than eliminate it.

Whether as patient or therapist, if we rush toward certainty prematurely, we run the risk of acting more out of ungrounded impulses than out of solid intuition. We act *impulsively* if we attempt to move away from, foreshorten, or shut down difficult experience of some sort, such as emotional pain, the confusion of not-knowing, or the challenge to dwell in ambiguity. We act *intuitively* when we remain fully open to whatever experience is before us, no matter how it feels and no matter how much ambiguity or uncertainty we might face. During psychotherapy it can be difficult to tell the difference between these two modes of response—impulsive versus intuitive. One clue to the difference involves the sense of urgency. When we feel pressured or desperate to make an intervention, as if needing to "discharge" it, short of life-threatening circumstances, we are more likely to be acting out of impulse than out of intuition. We are likely to be running with our discomfort than learning how to sit still in the midst of it. With Gus, as with all patients, we continually dance on this line between impulse and intuition.

When the mind/body/brain is treated as a single unified system, then health and well-being cannot be separated from the quality of our relationships, including self-other relations as well as self-self connections (Marks-Tarlow, 2008a), to the core of our own emotional selves. From this more complex broad-scale vantage point, not only physical conditions but especially problems addressed in psychotherapy cannot always be clearly defined, much less their solutions. From the start, my communication with Gus was filled with twists, turns, and potential land mines. Gus kept asking for what I intuitively sensed he did not need and could not use. Twice I took the risk of saying "no" rather than gratifying his requests: first, by refusing to help him evacuate a primary aspect of self; second, by refusing to diagnose him immediately. Rather than to reject me for it, Gus actively and willingly kept engaging with me. Consciously he wanted one thing; unconsciously he responded to another.

From my end, Gus's requests triggered strong visceral reactions. The implicit level of my body protested loudly and clearly from the start. On the phone my gut contracted at Gus's rejection of such a vital part of his inner experience. During our first session my jaw clamped down and my mouth refused to cooperate when asked for an immediate diagnosis. The more I responded to the implicit level in Gus, the more implicitly he sensed the safety net I offered. A similar pattern was repeated again and again throughout our work. Over time I came to understand these implicit exchanges more consciously, to see how they served to protect Gus from his own self-destructive urges and tendencies to implode.

To the degree that implicit and explicit processes possess distinct neurobiological underpinnings, everyone experiences a gap between these different levels. Yet there was more than a gap in Gus; there was a deep schism inside that at times felt more like a war. From the start I intuitively sensed great complexity regarding Gus's presenting issue. While uncertain as to the details, I could tell we would need lots of time for true clarity to emerge. I also sensed that in order to arrive at Gus's inner truths we both needed the courage to dive into unchartered waters. From my end, this was a case without precedent or preconception, forcing me to feel my way through by intuition alone. No set formula would prove as useful as my own careful attunement to Gus's current states in conjunction with my own inner world.

INTUITION IN LIFE AND DEATH
CIRCUMSTANCES

Within the cognitive literature there is ample research showing that implicit memory and learning work best in contexts such as I have just described for Gus, characterized by high degrees of complexity, ambiguity, or uncertainty (Claxton, 1997). Perhaps there is not enough information to make a reason-based decision. Or there may be so much complexity that it becomes impossible to parse the situation into component elements. Or precise circumstances might remain unknown, yet we still have to act anyway. Within psychotherapy the call to respond can get especially poignant during pivotal moments of crisis, danger, or upheaval.

When we are pressed to perceive, understand, and act under such conditions, left-brain deliberation is less useful partly because it operates in a vacuum compared to right-brain intuition (McGilchrist, 2009). The left brain is primarily connected to the body through the voluntary muscle system. By contrast, the right brain goes deep into the body's sensory, limbic, and autonomic nervous system (Schore, 1994, 2003a, 2003b). Left-brain deliberation pursues abstraction by cleaving the general case from particular details. In this way left-brain logic is designed to strip away all contexts. Right-brain awareness is more holistic partly through remaining fully immersed in context.

Within clinical work the context includes our own bodies, which are themselves submerged in an emotional, relational context with our patients whose details and dynamics shift unceasingly from moment to moment. By belonging to the implicit realm, clinical intuition is more akin to a mindless body than to a disembodied mind. When the body learns and remembers, it does so in context through direct experience. The nonconscious body appears to have a mind of its own in contrast to the conscious mind, which is attempting to learn facts. The latter requires deliberate focus, effort, and concentration, while implicit learning is automatic, rapid, and effortless (Claxton, 1997).

Complex, uncertain, and ambiguous circumstances are precisely the conditions that fit the field of critical-care nursing. Critical-care nurses manage patients with life-threatening problems that require complex assessment, high-intensity therapies and interventions, and continuous nursing vigilance. Patients may be unconscious and unable to articulate distress or changes in internal function. In order to anticipate patient needs, nurses must be attuned to tiny signals connected to physiological processes that often change rapidly and unexpectedly. Failure to read a shift or a wrong decision made in response can easily prove fatal.

A body of research surrounds the value of clinical intuition within the field of critical nursing (Benner, Hooper-Kyriakidis, & Stannard, 1999; Benner & Tanner, 1987; Brokensha, 2002, Cioffi, 1997; Effkin, 2001; Gerrity, 1987; King & Appleton, 1997; Lamond & Thompson, 2000; Pellegrino, 1979; Rew, 1986; Rew & Barron, 1987; Young, 1987). Discussion even touches on precognitive capacities to sense critical shifts in patients before they happen (Rew & Barron, 1987). Yet even in a field that advocates for clinical intuition, the topic generally remains highly charged. A tug-of-war exists regarding the validity of clinical intuition compared with evidence-based approaches. For example, Lamond and Thompson (2000) argued that evidence-based approaches help avoid *bad clinical judgment* in the form of *automatic biases* during intuitive decision making.

A long and distinguished tradition revolves around cognitive research that examines automatic biases during decision making. Daniel Kahneman, a psychology professor at Princeton University, located intuitive judgments between the automatic operations of perception and the deliberate operations of reasoning. In 2002 Kahneman received a Nobel Prize for his contributions to economics (there are no Nobel Prizes for psychology). During his acceptance speech, Kahneman underscored how even "people who know better" cannot help themselves when under the influence of "flawed intuitions," thus suggesting that automatic thinking is inferior to deliberate reasoning.

This was certainly the case in Kahneman's first study (Tversky and Kahneman, 1971), which investigated how experienced researchers make statistical judgments. Kahneman employed exactly the sort of experimental conditions in which logic and deliberate reasoning work best. These conditions are illustrated by the following example. For the full effects, try solving the problem before reading on.

A bat and a ball cost $1.10 in total.

The bat costs $1 more than the ball.

How much does the ball cost?

Most of us have an initial instinct to answer "10 cents," because the sum $1.10 separates naturally into $1 and 10 cents and 10 cents is close to the right amount. Kahneman (2002) cited statistics that many intelligent people yield to this immediate impulse: 50% (47/93) of Princeton students and 56% (164/293) of students at the University of Michigan answered incorrectly.

A little more deliberation brings the correct answer of 5 cents. But notice the context surrounding the study itself. A clear set of parameters exists. There is nothing ambiguous in the question posed to subjects. Not only is the problem clearly defined with a single correct answer, but the experimental setup was actually devised to throw us off so as to pit reason against intuition with stacked odds. The design of the study itself leaves no room for any other conclusion: People who use deliberate reason appear superior to those who rely on impressionistic approaches.

Certainly there is a time and a place for careful, conscious deliberation, especially when solving math problems. But returning to the job of the critical-care nurse, accuracy may be paramount, but timing is just as critical. In a triage situation or medical emergency, there may be little opportunity to carefully weigh options or double-check reasoning. In contrast to math problems these are not abstract dilemmas posed in neutral environments with leisurely time for cross-checks. The lives of very real patients often depend on concrete responses delivered as rapidly as possible. What is more, the high responsibility and potential lethal consequences create a highly emotionally charged context. The necessity for vigilant monitoring, attuned care taking, and quick responses under conditions of high arousal falls closer to the purview of parental intuition, a topic explored in greater detail in the chapter to come.

A TIME FOR EVERYTHING

Guy Claxton (1997), a psychologist, detailed three different processing speeds of the mind/brain/body system. The first and evolutionarily oldest level is the very fast processing speed of physical or body intelligence, or what some people refer to as our "wits." The middle processing speed relates to conscious thought, deliberation, strategy, and planning. The slowest processing speed involves insight that emerges from unconscious sources and incubation according to its own timetable. Whereas fast body intelligence and slow creative simmering are both right-brain processes, the middle speed of conscious thought is a product of the left brain. All three modes have their place in clinical work, and we continually shuttle back and forth between all three.

When we are immersed in the thick of things with patients, it is this fast processing physical intelligence that continually scans and updates our readings of our patients and ourselves. We share this type of implicit processing with animals, and it originates in subcortical areas of the brain (e.g., the brain stem, hypothalamus, amygdala, and insula), which are well beneath the thinking part of the brain or cerebral cortex. Body intelligence supports the sensory and emotional core of the embodied self, as connected to our very survival instincts.

That the body has a mind of its own is particularly evident when emotions run extremely high. Whether the emergency is real (outer world derived) or imagined (inner world perceived), a response is required but there is little time to think or make decisions. Imagine that you are sitting with a patient who suddenly jumps out of his chair in rage. He rushes at you with a knife. What do you do? Do you grab the knife, run away, reach for the phone, or scream loudly? Whatever you imagine under neutral conditions of reading this scenario is only a matter of speculation. The context is too far removed from the highly charged environment of the actual scene to predict with any accuracy. This is precisely why, with highly traumatized or dysregulated patients, it is so important to work at the edges and not squarely in the center of the regulatory boundaries (Ogden et al., 2009; Schore, 2009a). The body comes alive under conditions of high arousal in very different ways than under conditions of low or medium arousal.

During my graduate student days just a week before defending my dissertation thesis, I attended a dance performance in a seedy section of Los Angeles. During intermission I stood outside in an alley with two friends. A car pulled up next to us. A man aimed a gun through the open window, demanding our money and valuables. What I did was to turn around and run as fast as I could from that gun. Had I been asked my prediction before the incident, I would have guessed without hesitation that I would stay put and hand over my wallet. With my actual behavior such a complete surprise, I now understand why, in the heat of the moment, some people unexpectedly become heroes while others cannot live up to their own bravado.

William James picked up on this rapid level of implicit intelligence in 1884 in a seminal article called "What Is an Emotion." Published in a philosophical journal called *Mind* in the days before psychological journals existed, James had this query: When faced with a bear in the woods, do we run because we are afraid or are we afraid because we run? Based on our own subjective experience, most of us would reply that we run because we are afraid. This makes most sense to the conscious, rational mind, which loves to create narratives where deliberation, choice, and willpower play starring roles.

Yet from the perspective of the neuroscientist Benjamin Libet (Libet & Kosslyn, 2004) our subjective experience is only fiction if we look closely at brain processes. Here is the actual sequence according to what Libet calls "brain time." First the amygdala detects the bear and registers fear, which takes less than half a second. This triggers the nearly instantaneous subcortical responses in the basal ganglia and cerebellum to initiate the motor response of running, which also occurs in less than half a second. Only later do we consciously register what happened and how we feel about it, drawing on cortical responses that take longer than half a second. The amygdala, a subcortical part of the limbic or emotion-processing aspect of the brain (see Figure 2.1), is specialized for fear and is online at birth. Unlike other higher-level limbic structures, the amygdala does not need learning or any postnatal experience to register and respond to this kind of mortal danger. It is easy to see the evolutionary value of this kind of rapid, automatic processing.

Implicit processes take over in emergencies, and yet they are automatically and continually "on" all the time, scanning and responding to our social and physical environments at levels beneath our conscious awareness. That we continually scan and respond to our physical environments is clear when we drive our cars on autopilot. We start dreaming about that vacation we are planning only to look up and realize we just missed our turn. From the vantage point of memory, this kind of body intelligence is also called procedural memory, because it involves learning physical procedures or a sequence of actions (e.g., first we put our foot on the brake, then we shift into gear, step on the gas, and so forth). Being on autopilot combined with the term "procedural" could imply a robotic kind of intelligence.

While this is sometimes the case, procedural memory and implicit processes are also involved in the highest degrees of skill. Just listen to Rimsky-Korsakov's "Flight of the Bumblebee." You will get a sense of how the pianist's hands move at speeds much faster than conscious thought could ever dictate. That we register a continual stream of sensations, perceptions, and emotions is also evident within the body-to-body encoun-

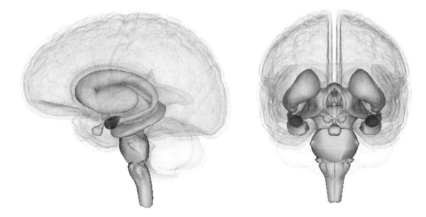

Figure 2.1. A side and front view of the amygdala (indicated bilaterally in black), which is the brain and body's most basic register of emotion. During psychotherapy, this subcortical structure is central to rapid implicit processing. As the most primitive arbiter of safety, danger plus the emotional sense of salience, the amygdala is online from the start of life, giving even newborns keen awareness of how they feel within their social environments. (From Anatomography, website maintained by Life Science Databases [LSDB])

ters mediated through body language. Whether or not we consciously tune in to our perceptions and feelings, as mentioned earlier we continually register and broadcast our reactions to the world around us implicitly through gestures and facial expressions.

Consider the plight of a male patient who is married to a high-powered business executive. This woman continually yawned when talking to her husband, sometimes as many as 15 times during a brief conversation. From my patient's perspective, through body language, his wife continually expressed boredom and a lack of interest in him. This became excruciatingly painful when amplified by the woman's consistent lack of empathy for his point of view. My patient's wife appeared to be out of touch with her body and unable to get beyond its literal expression during her insistence that she was right: To her, a yawn meant that she was tired and nothing more. This rendered it preposterous, even narcissistic, for her husband to think her body was making a social statement about his value to her.

In general we cannot control much of what we broadcast through body language. A highly observant person who is trained to understand facial musculature can tell the difference between a fake smile, which only engages the voluntary muscles surrounding the mouth, and a real smile, which also engages the involuntary muscles surrounding the eyes. These fast-moving body signals provide clues into underlying emotional experience, which we register and process underneath the surface of ongoing conscious awareness.

THE GIST OF CLINICAL INTUITION

With this information about implicit processes and right-brain awareness in mind, let us now return to the field of critical-care nursing to see how various researchers have characterized clinical intuition:

- Understanding without rationale (Benner & Tanner, 1987);
- Immediate knowledge of something without the conscious use of reason (Schraeder & Fischer, 1987);
- Lacking underlying conscious processes, not being able to be explained in a tangible manner (Cioffi, 1997);
- Knowing something about the patient that cannot be verbalized, that is verbalized with difficulty, or for which the source of knowledge cannot be determined (Young, 1987);
- Knowledge of a fact or truth, as a whole; immediate possession of knowledge; and knowledge independent of the linear reasoning process (Rew, 1986);
- A perception of possibilities, meanings, and relationships by way of insight; the sudden perception of a pattern in a seemingly unrelated series of events, beyond what is visible to the senses (Gerrity, 1987);
- The integration of forms of knowing in a sudden realization, which then precipitates an analytical process that facilitates action in patient or client care (King & Appleton, 1997);
- The ability to experience the elements of a clinical situation as a whole, to solve a problem or reach a decision with limited concrete information (Schraeder & Fischer, 1986);
- Three themes such as cognitive inference (rapid unconscious processing of cues), gestalt intuition (gaps of data filled in to complete a pattern), and precognitive function (perceiving a change before it happens) (Rew, 1988); and
- Key aspects of intuitive judgment, including pattern recognition, similarity recognition, commonsense understanding, skilled know-how, sense of salience, and deliberative rationality (Dreyfus & Dreyfus, 1986).

From this list, I have fleshed out five recurrent characteristics:

- Sudden recognition;
- Immediate knowledge;

- Emergent awareness;
- Nonverbal insight; and
- Holistic, integrative sensibilities.

The remainder of this chapter illustrates each characteristic with a representative case example.

Sudden Recognition

Once in a while psychotherapy involves smooth transitions accompanying major insight but most of the time the process involves messy stumbling. Freud's "royal road" to enlightenment easily slips into Bromberg's "bumpy road" when disowned, dissociated pieces of our selves suddenly collide within the therapeutic process to open up new realms of experience. Clinical intuition involves sudden recognition partly because both insight and change during psychotherapy are nonlinear. It is not always easy to see where we have been, much less where we are going. Sometimes the process involves long stretches of barren periods or impasses followed by unpredictable turns and sudden insights. To illustrate this kind of process I present the case of Sabina, a young woman suffering deeply from a history of extreme abuse and trauma, with whom I have been working for years.

In Chapter 1, I shared Sabina's transference dream, where I was underwater and waving my arms as if holding paintbrushes, while the dead body of an adolescent boy drifted upward. That highly charged dream followed a long period when Sabina and I had drifted for months in a holding pattern. As opposed to the rich texture of previous and later stages, at that point sessions were feeling somewhat repetitive, as if the two of us were locked in a mutual stance of defensive disengagement. For me, frustration was slowly building at the sense of impasse until a session came that changed everything. On that particular day, Sabina described a dream unlike any other in my clinical experience.

I am back in my old house in India. The roof is knocked off. My mother is there. So is my daughter Maya [a 2-year-old toddler] who wanders off in search of a shoe. Suddenly I notice a tidal wave heading towards me. It's absolutely huge. The water is clear. I feel desperate to protect myself. I back up against the wall. From here I watch the wave approach. But while looking at this wave I don't realize there is another one coming from the opposite direction. The water is black and this second wave sweeps over the house. Water fills the room and rises and rises. I'm struggling for my life. But somehow I manage to make it through. Slowly the water recedes. Then I see my mother coming towards me. She's got Maya in her arms, holding her high in the air. Maya appears dead. Her body is limp. My mother thrusts my daughter towards me. She is snarling with an almost satisfied look of contempt on her face. I stare in horror.

This dream terrified Sabina who could not recall any other of this variety. This was nothing like her typical recurrent theme—being chased by monsters, relatives, or other scary people. Over the course of my clinical career, I have come to believe that recurrent dreams reflect the emotional landscape that goes all the way back to infancy, a kind of preverbal tone implicitly set by the quality of our early relationships. Sabina's usual recurrent dream of being chased and even killed by scary others makes perfect sense, given her highly traumatic history, which included sexual molestation by her father along with accusations of blame by her mother. But in this instance Sabina produced another sort of dream whose tidal wave imagery matched precisely *what I used to dream as a child*. Within my inner landscapes, sometimes a giant tsunami would slowly approach and wash over me, occasionally while I was backed against a wall. Sometimes I was already in the water, alone or communally, with furniture floating all around the people. I never died, and these dreams were not always unpleasant. Sometimes they were even comical. The frequency of such dreams peaked during middle childhood when my parents were often out at night or traveling abroad for weeks with little contact. I was filled with abandonment fears and had great difficulty falling asleep at night. Frequently I awoke in terror.

When Sabina recounted her dream, it touched a place deep inside me—a place previously asleep for years. A sensory-based, full-body memory suddenly swept over me. Instantly I had vivid images of how terrified I used to feel as a little girl, especially at night. I remembered sucking my thumb and rocking. I remembered images of my parents going out amid fears they would never come back. I remembered calculations of how old I would be if I lost them at what age, and what age maybe I would feel safe if only I could make it there.

Along with all this embodied experience came a sudden recognition regarding this case. Over these past several months I had been subtly aloof. Sabina had been expressing jealousy toward other woman along with other insecurities. I had noticed myself feeling mildly irritated, but I had brushed off the significance. In this instant I suddenly understood how my own insensitivities had been playing into the picture. By brushing off my own discomforts I was also brushing off Sabina's. My blocked empathy had only exacerbated Sabina's experience of isolation and desperation.

The psychoanalyst Susan Sands proposed that, within psychotherapy, dreams sometimes "activate powerful forms of unconscious affective communication between patient and analyst, which crucially facilitate the transformation of dissociative mental structure" (2011, p. 357). Sabina's dream appeared to emerge from the relational unconscious on a mission to "seek and find" a deeper connection with me so as to open up greater channels of empathy. Indeed, Sabina's dream helped me attune to my role in our impasse by seeing where our interior worlds overlapped and where I had erected defenses against painful memories. I now saw how I had enacted the emotionally withholding mother in part who was shaming and blaming her daughter for her failures (I had recently called Sabina's attention to the fact that she had hardly mentioned her 2-year-old daughter in months). I also saw how I had enacted the child in part who was upset at her mother's neglect (I now understood my previous irritation with Sabina as a defense to ward off rousing my underlying abandonment fears).

Sands suggested that implicit-level dream communication is particularly likely to occur when overwhelming experience is dominating treatment. Indeed, Sabina's dream came just as a major crisis was erupting involving her daughter (recently diagnosed with autism following my suggestion for evaluation). In the weeks that followed, a torrent of ruptures and resolutions broke loose, as evidenced by the transference dream discussed earlier. This was a scary time. Suicidal feelings arose. Sabina even stopped eating at one point. She had grown utterly hopeless. Her life hung on a frayed line. Bonds of trust stretched thin between us.

Fortunately through communicating directly from one unconscious to another, Sabina's dream helped to restore my fuller experience of compassion. Although this period was excruciatingly painful for us, we each withstood the massive waves of emotion that followed. Once the torrent of intense emotion passed, we were brought to a new level of trust. In the process, a higher level of complexity emerged in Sabina, who felt less wounded and more compassionate toward the shortcomings of others. This newfound sense of resilience enabled Sabina to reconnect with her mother after many years of estrangement.

Immediate Knowledge

In the case of Sabina, while insight was sudden, it was not immediate. Our work during psychotherapy had reached an impasse that had extended for months. The breakthrough was grueling and a long time coming. The next example involves immediate knowledge that took no time at all to arrive during the fifth session of psychotherapy, when a 13-year-old named Stu brought his first dream into psychotherapy:

My friend Chantelle and I are going to a party. Lots of Greek gods and other fairytale figures are also invited. I know them all, but can't remember all their names. But it's easy to recognize Pinocchio. He's staring at me with his laser-beam, beady black eyes. Then he begins to follow me. I'm feeling uncomfortable. I find Chantelle and tell her it's time to leave the party. Then the scene switches. We are in Macy's. We're hiding in the clothes under one of the racks. We hang out there for a while. Then I get bored and want to come out.

Stu is a very verbal, highly creative adolescent who easily associated with various dream elements:

- Greek gods: *As a little kid I loved to hear and read stories about Greek gods. I spent lots of time playing out their stories in fantasy. At first I would play-act the different figures. As I grew older I would tell their tales out loud as if speaking to an invisible audience.*
- Forgetting the characters' names: *I know exactly what that is. Do you remember that musical I just tried out for? Well, I didn't make any of the main characters, because I screwed up the audition. I forgot some of the words to my song. I've never done that before. It was really embarrassing . . .*
- Hiding out in a Macy's clothes rack: *A couple of weeks ago, Chantelle and I took a bus to West Hollywood (famous for its gay population). We had so much fun going into all the stores! We tried on lots of wigs, shoes, and crazy clothes.*

Upon hearing Stu's dream and even before he associated to its elements I *immediately knew* something was weighing on his mind. My intuition was ringing a bell to alert me: Either Stu's hiding something or he's really conflicted about talking about it, to the point of covering up. Despite my suspicion of exactly what this might be, I never count on certain knowledge without checking it out.

T: *Stu, I'm struck by that Pinocchio figure in your dream. That's the part that catches my attention—the way he's staring at you and following you. After leaving the party you wind up hiding in the store. All this makes me wonder if there's something going on for you that you may be hiding or that's hard to talk about.*

Stu: *Even though I'm really young and I know it's unusual, for a couple of years I've known I'm gay. I haven't talked about it with my mom and dad. But I don't think it will be all that hard for me to come out to my family. I have gay and lesbian relatives on both my mother's and my father's sides. Anyway I sort of hint at it and get the sense my parents already kind of know. But there's this other thing, this fantasy I've been having lately. It's kind of hard to talk about . . . but . . . I think I might want to become a drag queen . . . maybe as my future career. You know like Lady Bunny or RuPaul? But I'm really scared my parents won't go for this.*

While it was difficult to bring these issues up himself, Stu felt the freedom and safety to discuss them once I expressed interest and took the initiative to ask. He became quite animated after I "pulled" the information out of him. Stu didn't want the session to end. He liked me penetrating his dream symbolism and even expressed the desire for his parents to ask him more questions about his sexuality.

This session illustrated how an immediate hunch can guide clinical response. Instantly I knew something was up; all I had to do was check in about that. The rest was a collaborative effort. Because it arises and unfolds in a relational context, clinical intuition often works like this.

Nonverbal Insight

While they do include dialogue, dreams are primarily visual in nature. Most mammals dream. The human fetus spends much of its time in REM sleep, the stage in which dreams occur. Perhaps because dream images are such an early part of the nonverbal landscape, imagery is a central form of intuition. Clinical insight frequently takes a nonverbal form partly because, developmentally, a preverbal period precedes language and partly because so much communication occurs nonverbally in the first place. Even if we do not speak the same language as someone or share the same culture, Darwin (1872) revealed first, followed by Ekman (2003), how people the world over, along with other mammals (see Panksepp, 1998), broadcast their emotions through the musculature of their faces, their postures, and how they move their bodies (see Figure 2.2).

That clinical insight often begins in nonverbal form is well illustrated by the following case, reported by the psychoanalyst Thomas Arizmendi in 2008. The patient was a single, depressed woman in her mid-thirties who claimed to enter psychotherapy as a last resort, the only alternative to suicide. In retrospect, Arizmendi interpreted these words as a dissociated aspect of this woman's self desperately in search of a safe environment in which to become known. The woman's history of severe trauma resulted in extended silences during therapy, when she would sit hunched over, her long hair covering her face. Arizmendi described a pervasive sense of deadness in the room. Words had no place there. Every attempt to reach the patient through interpretations was rebuffed as meaningless and irrelevant. So much for the royal road to enlightenment as attained through the classical psychoanalytic methods.

Feelings of helplessness and aloneness consumed the therapist. He could feel his own body along with that of his patient's driven into paralyzed retreat. Yet simultaneously Arizmendi sensed something more active within the very deadness, as if his own sensibilities represented a communication from the patient about how she felt during her early life attendant to trauma. Arizmendi came to liken his paralysis to times when his patient's father would enter her bedroom late at night, leading her to collapse into a disoriented, lifeless-like posture as she held her breath.

As the sessions progressed, the patient became increasingly fearful that she had been sexually abused. Increasingly, paper and pen became a

PLATE III

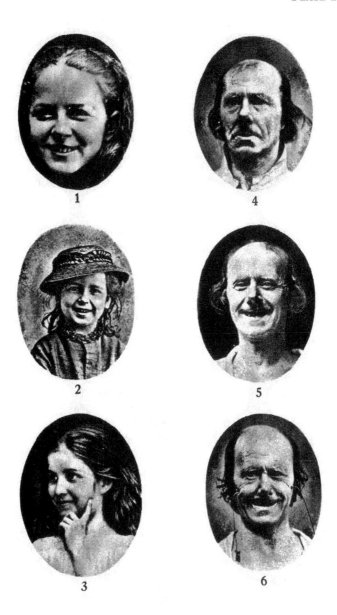

Figure 2.2. Plate III from *The Expression of the Emotions in Man and Animals* by Charles Darwin, originally published in 1872. This plate was drawn from Chapter VIII, which discussed joy, high spirits, love, tender feelings, and devotion.

medium of meaningful communication between herself and her therapist. The patient would furiously grab the pen often with her fist in a process so reflexive and primitive that at one point she drew spectacularly with her left hand despite being right-handed, a fascinating detail on which Arizmendi spent quite a bit of time speculating.

As the drawings progressed, entering therapy in bits and pieces over time, so did the insights. At one point the patient recognized an L-shaped object as the faucet of her bathtub threatening to touch her backside if she did not carefully watch it whenever bathing. Meanwhile, Arizmendi described his own "feeble, ineffective" efforts to "see" what she was communicating by "cognitively" attempting to make sense of the pictures. Whenever he operated using conscious thought like this, Arizmendi noticed a kind of disconnect between patient and therapist, as if they were operating on separate but parallel levels, revealed by their disjointed verbal exchanges.

Then one day something else happened when Arizmendi let go of all intellectual attempts to figure things out. The patient had drawn what looked to her like a big rug, but she could not understand one puzzling feature of her own drawing. She kept wondering why the lines did not meet at one corner, on the lower right (see Figure 2.3a). Arizmendi noticed a sense of gloominess washing over the room, followed by a feeling of doom and he simply surrendered to his experience. From within this atmosphere an image then came to him of two electrical wires that touched to create a jolt inside of his body. Arizmendi reflected, "Maybe you don't have them meet because that's where the disaster is!"

The patient instantly grabbed her pen with her fist plus a clean sheet of paper. She furiously began scribbling chaotic lines with heavy pressure,

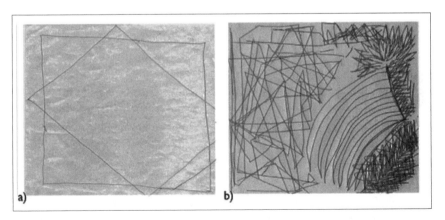

Figure 2.3. (a) Patient drawing made before the therapist's "disaster" comment; (b) Patient drawing made after the therapist's "disaster" comment. (Courtesy of Thomas Arizmendi)

including stabbing right through the paper in the same corner (see the lower right-hand corner of Figure 2.3b). The unanticipated shock was barely containable that session. During the next several weeks, this was accompanied by the patient's direct experience of what previously had been dissociated anger and rage. She had talked about the "fire in [her] stomach" and had even experienced it as a raw emotion. But she had never identified such feelings before as part of her complete self, one that carried affective meaning within the context of her actual history.

Clearly this is a case where a nonverbal method led to a nonverbal insight in the therapist that opened up a nonverbal flood of experience previously locked so deeply within the patient's body that words just would not suffice. In fact, words only served to drive direct experience away. In this case, which is so typical of early trauma and abuse, motoric actions, somatosensory symptoms, and intense affect states, rather than words, were how the patient "informed" the therapist of painful and often preverbal experiences. These nonverbal clues triggered an image in the therapist—of two electrical wires touching to create a jolt—which served as a metaphor to guide Arizmendi's response, ultimately facilitating the further release of dissociated emotion and arousal. This play of intuition through visual imagery and metaphor is a topic covered extensively in Chapter 6.

Emergent Awareness

Many clinical examples so far also illustrate emergent awareness, perhaps because emergent awareness is a hallmark of nonlinear change within psychotherapy. But here I will take this a step further by relaying what happened when I decided to write this book. After I chose the topic of clinical intuition, I became extraordinarily curious about the experiences of friends and colleagues. I started asking around for clinical stories I might include in these pages. This next one came from a female psychoanalyst I met at the 2010 Congress of Neuropsychoanalysis in Seattle.

To set the stage for her story, the psychoanalyst first described the layout of her office, which was separated from her waiting room by a very long hall. One day after picking up a patient from the waiting room, she was walking down the hall behind him, until he turned the corner into her office where she could no longer see him. As the man sat down, she heard him let out a long and highly audible sigh that immediately conjured up an ominous thought within her: "Oh no! I hope I won't have to do CPR on him."

After the therapist entered her office and the session began, the man immediately told her the story of what a difficult week it had been. He and a really good friend had gone to play basketball. While playing, the friend suddenly collapsed onto the floor. He was not moving and had lost consciousness. The woman's patient tried to give his friend CPR to resuscitate him, but it did not work. The paramedics could not help either. In the prime of his life and with no history or previous warning of illness, the patient's friend died.

Understandably the man's psychoanalyst was flabbergasted, not only at the story itself, which was shocking enough, but also at her own ability to have detected its gist ahead of time. What was it about the sound of her patient's sigh that conjured up the image of administering CPR? How did this awareness emerge? This story either gives someone the chills (which is what happened to me—as I listened, I felt goosebumps rising on my arms), or it can raise someone's cackles (no wonder so many researchers and theoreticians have avoided the topic of clinical intuition—to get away from examples such as these!).

When I began this project I was fully aware that clinical intuition had been avoided as a legitimate topic of scientific interest partly out of the myth that it involves magic or that it works through mysticism. I was keenly aware of the existence of medical intuitives—people who diagnose and treat physical ailments and mental suffering through intuition alone, without the benefit of background medical information or diagnostic tests. I had read the work of Carolyn Myss (1997), a famous medical intuitive who was visited and read by thousands. I had attended a talk given by Judith Orloff, a Western trained psychiatrist so taken by the predictions and accuracy of her intuition that she ultimately blended traditional and alternative healing approaches. Orloff (2010) described early either/or struggles between the established perspectives and techniques of Western science versus the inner tugs of her own intuitive wisdom.

Despite a personal interest in these subjects, I nonetheless intended to stay away from them in this book. Because I wanted to rescue clinical intuition from the closet, I wanted to re-establish the scientific legitimacy of the topic. Yet people shared too many stories like the one above, so I could not stay away from these topics completely in all due conscience. Besides, in my heart of hearts, I firmly believe there is a firm scientific grounding for all acts of intuition, no matter how remarkable they may seem. This belief is partly reflected in my last book, *Psyche's Veil*, which presents the holistic paradigm of nonlinear science as a framework for integrating the science, art, mythology, and spirituality of psychotherapy (Marks-Tarlow, 2008a).

Holistic, Integrative Sensibilities

The world looks very different when perceived from linear versus nonlinear perspectives. When we don linear lenses, complex wholes can be broken down into component parts. The parts can be examined and understood independently from one another, and then these separated understandings can be linked again into an integrated whole. Within psychotherapy, this might translate into approaching a complex clinical presentation by diagnosing component symptoms and then approaching the treatment of each symptom one by one. For example, a patient seeks help from a psychiatrist, with presenting complaints of being overweight and depressed. Given that the patient is not interested in long-term psychotherapy, the psychiatrist understandably may prescribe a diet to the woman, while sending her to Weight Watchers, simultaneously instructing her to engage in vigorous exercise as well as to take an antidepressant medication. The expectation is that by addressing each of these problems individually and systematically, this lady will feel better quickly as a whole (see Figure 2.4).

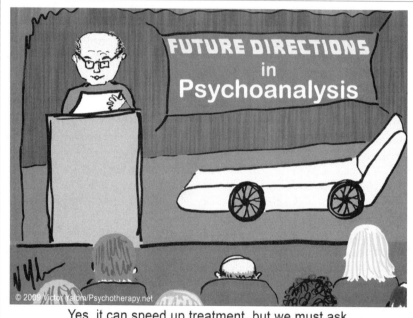

Yes, it can speed up treatment, but we must ask, "What are the transference implications?"

Figure 2.4. One reason that therapists treat patients in piecemeal fashion, as a collection of symptoms, is pressure for ever speedier treatments. From the perspective of minimizing costs and maximizing resources, this is understandable. Yet there is increasing evidence that the therapeutic bond is the fulcrum for deep, emotional healing underneath surface symptoms. In order to effect change that permeates the body and not just the mind, there is often no way around long-term psychotherapy. (2011 Victor Yalom/Psychotherapy.net)

From a nonlinear perspective, this sort of piecemeal approach can appear preposterous—like dissecting a living body into pieces in order to understand the connective tissue. At times, processes of reductive analysis not only alter but actually destroy the very phenomena one is trying to understand. At the beginning of this chapter I selected Gus's case partly to illustrate how this can be so. Gus's initial desire to be diagnosed worked hand in hand with hopes of ridding himself of a vital aspect of his core experience. To have gratified this side of his desires did not serve him. What served him better was to understand the destructive nature of his very urges.

Fortunately, each clinician (and person at large) has the synthetic workings of intuitive faculties to complement the piecemeal and fragmenting style of our analytic side. Within psychotherapy, the holistic lens provided by intuition helps us to perceive the big picture so that we may gain an overview of what is happening. In contrast to the linear perspective where the whole is made up of parts, the nonlinear perspective reverses things completely. When a system is highly complex, its parts are interdependent and inseparable from the workings of the whole. The result is that within highly complex systems (like relational dynamics within psychotherapy) *the whole becomes evident within the parts* instead. At the biological level, this is easy to see, when we consider that the entire genetic code for our bodies exists intact within each and every cell of our body. At the psychological level, this follows the common clinical lore that the whole of a session is apparent within the first exchange during the clinical hour, while the whole course of psychotherapy is apparent within the first clinical hour. As an example of this, consider the following clinical vignette.

When Suzette entered my office for the first time, this tiny, perky young lady actually jiggled as she walked through the door from my waiting room—half with nerves, half with excitement. Suzette flopped down on the couch, exclaiming, "I've never done this before. I don't know why I'm so nervous. I know I can talk about anything I want to in here. I know that it's confidential. So there's no reason to lie or worry about what other people think."

"I'm struck by your choice of words here, Suzette. You mentioned lying. Is that something you do often?"

"Actually I'm lying all the time right now. In fact, my whole life feels like a lie. I'm here because I just got arrested for prostitution, and I'm really freaked out. I came to Los Angeles from the Midwest with a big dream. I was a total star in my hometown. I was convinced that my combination of talent and determination was unstoppable and would cut through anything. I wanted to become an actress. When I came out to visit a year ago, I had a glorious day. The sun was shining. Everything looked bright, including my future. But then after I actually got here, everything started to go wrong. All I seemed to do was to wait in lines. I felt herded around like cattle. Pretty soon, I'd burned through all my money. I guess I got pretty desperate. Someone told me about this way to give massages with 'just a little twist at the end.' Suddenly this brought in a lot of money for a little work. I didn't have to take my clothes off; I never considered it prostitution. But when I found myself busted and in a courtroom, it was so humiliating to be looked at with so much contempt by that judge. As if I was some kind of vermin. I'm still in shock. How did I get here? What if my parents knew? But actually, no one knows about it at all. Except you—I can't believe you pulled this out of me in the first five minutes of being here."

"And how is it for you that I did that?"

"I feel really relieved. It's been so hard to hold that secret alone."

Suzette cried a lot, and she experienced much relief at admitting all the shame she had been bottling up. Her trance was broken. Recent events plus hearing herself talk about what happened cut through Suzette's denial about what she had been doing and how she had become caught up in her own lies. When Suzette returned the next session, and I brought up this instance, she admitted thinking to herself, "What am I, a piece of glass you can see right through?' I started shaking inside, wondering if everyone else can see through me like that? Do they all know these things about me?"

Over many sessions we discussed how what started off as tiny ways that she had kept things to herself around relatives to prevent them from "picking at her" had turned to a full-blown habit of keeping up a façade, with many people telling her they are unable to read how she feels, especially when she gets angry.

"It's a really slippery line between hiding from others and hiding from yourself. Like telling yourself you aren't *really* doing anything wrong by adding a little *twist* at the end of your massages, but then feeling dirty when others see it differently. I often get this squishy feeling in the pit of my stomach that I just want to ignore. When I'm alone I can ignore it much of the time by telling myself 'You're fine; you don't really need to deal with this.' But somewhere inside I know I *do* need to deal with it, and that everything really *isn't* okay."

From a nonlinear perspective, the whole of things is always present in the parts and pieces of experience. There is nothing magic about that. Suzette's whole truth was coiled up in the tiniest level of the musculature in her face, the stance of her body, and her choice of words. By hiding from others, Suzette eventually became hidden from herself, ignoring her own intuitive truths and choosing what she wanted to believe instead. Yet at an implicit level, she was still broadcasting the truth outward. We need only to look with the right intuitive lenses to detect the whole of things, even within the tiniest parts. Richard Feynman, the late Nobel Prize–winning physicist, once remarked, "Nature uses only the longest threads to weave her patterns, so each small piece of her fabric reveals the organization of the entire tapestry." While the fabric and threads are of interest in their own way, this book concerns the tapestry as a whole.

WRAP-UP

Clinical intuition involves implicit processes that lead us to know, feel, and sense things without knowing how we know. Stories abound of people intuitively sensing the distress, catastrophic accidents, or impending deaths of those who are close to their hearts. Lest we puff up with pride at our superhuman powers, such tales are not restricted to people. Tales also abound of house pets cowering under sofas or in the corner and rodents fleeing in collective panic just moments before a natural disaster, such as an earthquake, strikes. Whether or not the reader ascribes to this transpersonal level of intuition is a personal affair. But if such things are possible they happen because our bodies' wits are so contextually sensitive as to embrace the enormity of the universe at large.

When learning, the body does so beneath the level of conscious awareness, automatically, in context, through bottom-up processes that emanate upward from basic emotional, sensory, and other bodily experiences. Implicit learning, memory, and insight are effortless and immediate. The body appears to have a mind of its own. Implicit processes are heightened by highly emotionally charged circumstances.

As clinicians, whether or not we are able to keep our wits about us when the going gets tough is one mark of expertise. During challenging moments, are we guided by intuition or driven by impulse? By engaging in practices such as those outlined below, we maximize our chances of being inspired by intuition instead of being pushed by impulse. When we are guided by intuition, we remain open, engaged, and privy to the whole context, both inside and outside our bodies. When we are driven by impulse, we engage defensively instead by trying to ward off some aspect of experience that becomes too difficult or painful to bear. While it is often difficult to distinguish intuition from impulse, intuition is fueled partly by safety and trust available through secure attachment.

In order to facilitate implicit learning and receive your body's intuitive messages, here are six ways to set the foundation.

- Practice focus: both single-pointed as well as diffuse attention. Whether through yoga, meditation, or quiet sitting, we train our inner demons by stilling the body and quieting the mind.
- Open up your receptivity to inner emotional, sensory, and body-based cues. Close your eyes and engage in deep breathing as an excellent way to refocus attention toward inner subjective experience.
- Develop a ritual for clearing, grounding, and consulting your own intuition. Some therapists use outer measures (e.g., touching the heart with one or both hands, lighting a candle, or burning sage in the office to clear the air). Other therapists use inner measures

like consulting with an inner guide to ground themselves before a new patient or when dealing with a difficult case. A third possibility is to look out of the window or toward a pleasant picture to break away from disengaged, trancelike states.

- Contact your own inner signals.
  a. During a session, if you become aware of feeling "urgency," "stop" in order to see.
  b. Practice paying attention to your body by checking out sensations at various times during each session. Note after the session what you have noticed. Get used to noticing without judging or analyzing.
  c. When you look back at a session, practice "seeing" without analyzing how the various parts fit into the whole; again this is a way to learn to flex that intuitive "muscle."
- Clarify your values as a clinician. What brings greatest meaning to your practice? What do you as a unique individual have to offer to your patients? What feeds you the most in the process?
- Set intentions for yourself. Setting intentions is different than setting goals. First, setting intentions focuses *on the process of how you approach something*, rather *than the outcome of what you get out of it*. Second, rather than pressuring yourself to reach a certain goal, setting intentions *reduces pressure* as it opens up the space of possibilities. An intention might be created in the form of one or two words—*healing, growing, empathizing, being fully present, being authentic.* Or an intention might take the form of a short phrase—*I want to sit patiently until I find clarity; I strive to set aside my own needs and agendas in service of clarifying those of my patients,* and so on.

The chapter to come explores developmental lenses of the mammalian attachment system, where clinical intuition merges with parental instincts we share with other animals to bond, love, and nurture our young.

CHAPTER 3

Empathic Roots

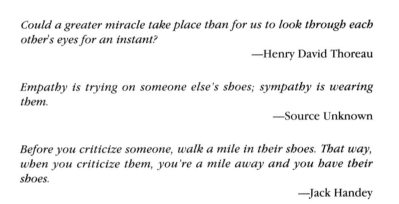

Could a greater miracle take place than for us to look through each other's eyes for an instant?

—Henry David Thoreau

Empathy is trying on someone else's shoes; sympathy is wearing them.

—Source Unknown

Before you criticize someone, walk a mile in their shoes. That way, when you criticize them, you're a mile away and you have their shoes.

—Jack Handey

W E BECOME PSYCHOTHERAPISTS OUT OF A desire to help others. In the process we often bear witness to intolerable suffering. Why do we gravitate toward such anguish and even relish the discomforts of our profession? Each therapist would give a different answer, depending on his or her distinct genetic, social, cultural and family background. I was my father's confidante. A colleague was a disabled sibling's advocate; another colleague was a drunken parent's caretaker. A host of implicit family mandates points us toward our calling. Yet despite these divergent histories, a common reason exists for why we become psychotherapists. At a primary embodied level, we all share the instinct to nurture and care for others as part of our psychoneurobiological wiring.

From an evolutionary standpoint, this wiring is ancient, dating back over 300 million years to the beginnings of mammals. Our reptilian predecessors laid large batches of eggs, leaving their young to play the odds and grapple with the elements, fight off predators, and generally fend for themselves. Mammals developed a new strategy for survival. They incubated fewer babies within their wombs, and then those babies were born in an immature, helpless state. This permitted open wiring and more neural plasticity in service of learning from experience.

Two main sets of social instincts—care of the young and the tendency to play—separate the open wiring of the mammalian brain from the closed wiring of the reptilian brain on which it sits. In the next chapter, I cover the topic of play; in the current chapter I relate clinical intuition to behavioral instincts to care for babies until maturity, while emotionally caring about what happens throughout life. During psychotherapy, in the heat of the moment, under the guidance of intuition, these relationally oriented instincts are what grab our bodies, stimulate our brains, and prompt our minds.

In the sections of this chapter, I explore the roots of clinical intuition within human empathy and the roots of human empathy within the mammalian attachment system. In order to illustrate how powerful and deep these ancient instincts are and how they bond us to fellow mammals, I next turn to a tale of animal intuition. From there, I launch into details about the neurobiology of empathy during human development. In order to illustrate these developmental processes with a human example, I describe the case of a woman whose early physical and sexual abuse interrupted her empathic connections to her own child.

INTERSPECIES KINDNESS

We humans love to pride ourselves on our differences from other animals. We are the only species to use multiple spoken languages, and we create books for our young and computers that interconnect our social and political existences across the globe. Yet these crowning glories also carry destructive power if we neglect the consequences of unbridled expansion upon other living creatures. While it is easy to privilege the power of left-brain higher-order thinking, the more we understand the centrality of emotion, the more our limbic circuitry can connect us to our fellow mammals. It is our mammalian core that lends humans the capacity for compassion and the courage to help others.

In all cultures, the hero is celebrated, honored, and valorized, both in myth and in life. The classic Western hero myth (see Campbell, 1949/1973) involves a knight in shining armor who fights a fierce dragon to rescue a damsel in distress. The universality of such myths attests to deeply rooted instincts to fight off predators and protect vulnerable others. This protective instinct also exists in animals. Most dog owners attest to how readily their pets provide warm nuzzles and affectionate licks when they display sorrow and grief. Steven Kotler, a dog rescuer, observed how empathy manifested in an older, unusually aggressive dog named Otis, a bull terrier and alpha dog of the pack:

> Otis outweighs Gidget by over sixty pounds, but to keep their matches even, he flops onto his back and fights with one paw. Rolling over and letting a smaller animal wrestle the "top" position is self-handicapping. Only using one paw is self-handicapping. But with Otis things go further. While he may fight with only one paw, Gidget fights with everything she's got—including her teeth. Occasionally she'll bite his face and not let go. When this happens, Otis likes to stand up and strut around, with Gidget dangling off him like a long furry earring. (2010, p. 125)

The psychotherapy community now capitalizes on animal empathy through programs such as equine therapy for victims of posttraumatic stress disorder and dolphin play for autistic children.

Along with tales of natural healing capacities and empathic instincts, animal rescue stories abound. The story I chose for this chapter involves a beluga whale named Mila who caught the world's attention in July 2009 when she saved the life of a drowning diver. The incident was captured on film during a free diving competition in China. The tank of water was more than 20 feet deep and chilled to arctic temperatures. The tank also included a group of whales there from the start in a Seaworld type of environment. Divers were instructed to hold their breath for as long as possible without the benefit of breathing equipment. A female competitor, Yang Yun, 26, was fine at first but then flew into a panic when sudden cramping paralyzed her legs, and she began to sink. The whales, having lots of experience with human divers, realized something had gone wrong. Mila went to Yun's rescue. In Figure 3.1a we see Mila maneuvering the diver with her mouth in order to right the woman's position. In Figure 3.1b, Mila takes hold of Yun's leg in order to lift her to the surface. In Yun's words, "I began to choke and sank even lower and I thought that was it for me—I was dead, until I felt this incredible force under me driving me to the surface."

Mila's response to Yun's predicament was remarkable, and her behavior was heroic. This whale of a tale is reminiscent of the story of Jonah and the whale from the Old Testament. After Jonah refused to fulfill God's wishes by going to Nineveh, God sent Jonah to sea in a boat, where he was thrown overboard, only to be rescued by a whale. After swallowing Jonah whole, the whale delivered him to dry land, after which Jonah completed God's bidding. Whether pointing regressively toward retreat or more progressively toward a spawning ground for Jonah's emotional development, the whale remains a poignant symbol for the womb.

In fact, a striking aspect of Mila's story is that both the whale and diver were female. Within our culture, the moral development of females often revolves around human needs, empathy, and interdependence, while the moral development of men involves individual rights plus abstract principles of right and wrong (Gilligan, 1982). That said, the issue of gender differ-

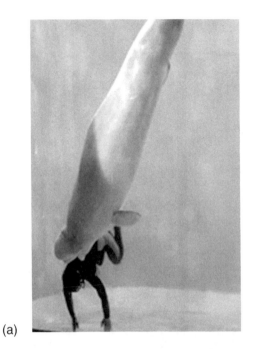

(a)

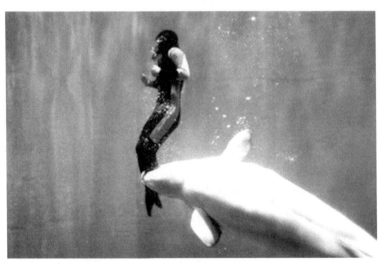

(b)

Figure 3.1. (a) Mila rights the diver; (b) Mila saves the diver from drowning. (Courtesy of Europics)

ences in empathy is controversial. All depends on how empathy is defined and how it is measured (see Eisenberg & Strayer, 1987). For example, women display greater empathy when measured by self-report, while less reliable differences are exhibited by physiological measures. One study (Rueckert & Naybar, 2008) found a correlation between right-hemisphere activation and empathy only in women. This suggests a possible neural basis for gender differences in empathy, which is supported by the finding that women are more likely than men to extend empathy to perceived enemies or competitors (Singer, Seymour, O'Doherty, Stephan, Dolan & Frith, 2006).

DISCRETE EMOTIONAL CIRCUITS

Certainly Mila was heroic, but did she display empathy toward the drowning diver? The issue of animal emotion as a felt experience is likewise controversial. Jaak Panksepp is a neuroscientist who studies ethology, the comparative science of animals, with a specialty in affective development. Although there is no way to prove through subjective report that other mammals experience feelings much like humans do, through the inclusion of evidence-based neuroscience, Panksepp certainly believes this to be the case (Panksepp, 2011; see Figure 3.2). He has written the definitive textbook in the field of comparative emotional development (Panksepp, 1998), based on studies of homologous (i.e., structurally similar) areas between animal and human limbic systems.

Beginning with the work of Darwin (1872) and continuing through to studies by Paul Ekman (2003), researchers' interest in the neurobiology of emotion has led them to examine discrete emotional circuits in the brain. Panksepp identified seven circuits that are common among all mammals: seeking, care, lust, play, panic, rage, and fear. Each has distinct neural architecture to link sensory, motivational, and behavioral areas of the brain. Yet an overlap exists in the neurochemical cocktail of excitatory and inhibitory transmitters released into synaptic gaps between neighboring neurons (see Figure 3.3). Glutamate, the most widespread excitatory neurotransmitter, works in tandem with GABA, its chemical precursor and the most widespread inhibitory neurotransmitter. Overlap also exists in how the circuits function. In humans, for example, lust melts into play during the dance of seduction and lust fuses with rage during the act of rape.

Panksepp's circuits link the layers identified by Paul MacLean in MacLean's concept of the triune brain (see Figure 3.4; MacLean, 1990). A reptilian layer serves as the foundation, related to reflex and survival needs. Overlaid on the reptilian layer is the mammalian limbic system, which introduces emotion and motivation to modulate basic needs. These two layers are then topped by the human neocortex, which permits the more conscious experiences of self-reflection, planning, and symbolic representation.

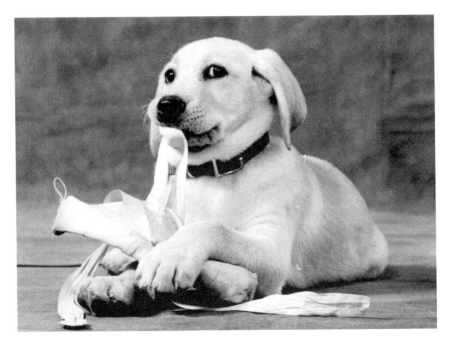

Figure 3.2. Whether dogs experience felt emotion as humans do is controversial to scientists. The problem is that animals cannot report on their subjective experience in the same way that humans can. Yet few dog owners would deny that their pets feel emotions. This dog named Lucky happened to get hold of her owner's ballet slipper. Does Lucky appear to be communicating emotion through her body language and facial expression? If so, what emotions can you read? (Courtesy of Benedicte Schoyen)

Of the three layers, the limbic system is the most interconnected layer. Each circuit extends downward into lower reptilian subcortical centers as well as upward into higher, uniquely human cortical areas. While the neocortex is necessary for emotional experience to reach full awareness, this area cannot generate feeling states. The subcortical origin of feelings means that animals probably do experience emotion but, from a fully immersed vantage point, without reflective awareness.

Within humans, as mentioned, both the expression and detection of emotion are specialties of the right hemisphere (McGilchrist, 2009; Schore, 1994), whose circuitry is lateralized to reach deep into the body's internal systems, partly through the interface between the limbic and autonomic nervous systems. Along with the enteric division, which helps us to digest food, the autonomic nervous system includes two branches. The

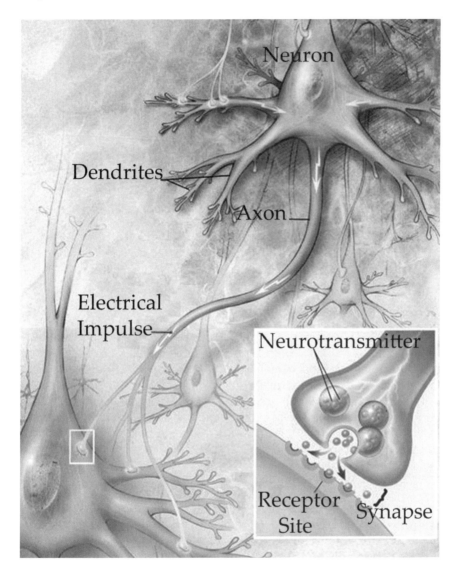

Figure 3.3. Here, the pathway of synaptic transmission is illustrated. The brain's neurochemistry is one key to its amazing complexity. Different neurotransmitters circulate through the same neural circuitry. This increases the brain's flexibility by boosting the number of potential states. (Public domain, U.S. National Institutes of Health, National Institute on Aging)

Triune Brain

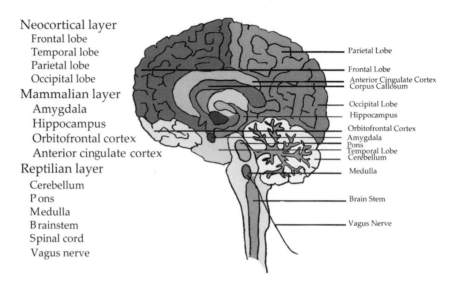

Neocortical layer
  Frontal lobe
  Temporal lobe
  Parietal lobe
  Occipital lobe
Mammalian layer
  Amygdala
  Hippocampus
  Orbitofrontal cortex
  Anterior cingulate cortex
Reptilian layer
  Cerebellum
  Pons
  Medulla
  Brainstem
  Spinal cord
  Vagus nerve

Parietal Lobe
Frontal Lobe
Anterior Cingulate Cortex
Corpus Callosum
Occipital Lobe
Hippocampus
Orbitofrontal Cortex
Amygdala
Pons
Temporal Lobe
Cerebellum
Medulla
Brain Stem
Vagus Nerve

Figure 3.4. This schematic of Paul MacLean's triune brain reveals the human brain in three layers, corresponding roughly to the onset of reptiles, mammals, and humans during evolution. Each layer sits atop lower levels, helping to regulate them while adding new functions. As with many subdivisions attributed to complex, biological systems, sharp boundaries between levels easily break down in what is ultimately indivisible circuitry. This is the case for the triune brain, which is more of a useful heuristic and metaphor than it is a technically accurate description. (Courtesy of the author)

sympathetic division up-regulates emotional arousal to deal with fight-or-flight panic or intense joy. The parasympathetic division down-regulates arousal to bring the body back to rest and relaxation (see Figure 3.5).

Whereas the reptilian layer matures in the womb, the mammalian social emotions mature after birth through a baby's interaction with primary caregivers. During the first two years life, through empathy, right-brain to right-brain communication between parents and children enables parents to sense and respond to their infants' emotional needs (see Schore, 2003a, 2003b). Empathically based communication occurs through non-verbal, subcortical channels using paralinguistic features like facial expression, tone and rhythm of voice, posture, and movements.

It makes sense that the higher limbic areas develop relationally. The broad function of emotion is relational. By assigning negative or positive valence to changes detected within inner and outer environments, emo-

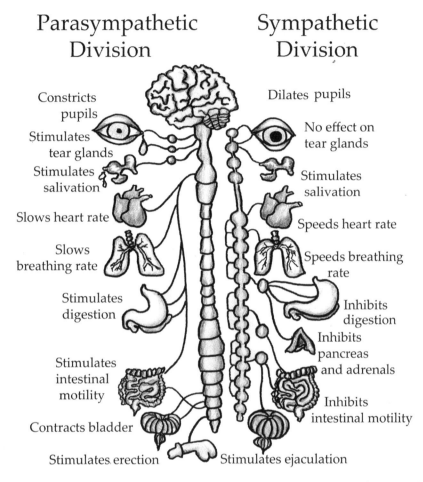

Figure 3.5. This shows a comparison between the sympathetic and parasympathetic branches of the autonomic nervous system. The sympathetic nervous system activates the fight-or-flight response by dilating the pupils, which promotes distance vision; increasing blood pressure and heart and breathing rates; and pumping blood toward the external muscles in preparation for immediate action. The parasympathetic nervous system promotes relaxation by constricting the pupils, which allows for closer vision; slowing down heart and breathing rates; and enhancing blood flow to the viscera and other internal organs, thereby promoting digestion and elimination. (Courtesy of the author)

tions help us to assess where we stand in relationship to our primary experience. There is a burgeoning trend in neuroscience away from cognition as a primary experience. Instead, researchers like Damasio, Fogel, Panksepp, and Schore now believe emotion rather than thought lies at the center of our highest human functions, including creativity, morality, meaning, and relationships.

Parental empathy, on which clinical intuition rests, derives primarily from the care circuit. Given that major aspects of our limbic circuitry mature in the first two years of life before we have words, language, and conscious thoughts, it is no wonder that clinical intuition rests on nonverbal, subcortical channels. This is how we sense, understand, and see patterns in and respond to the body-based states of our patients. Symbolic thought is important at points, including for insight and self-reflection. But emotion, both in unconscious and conscious as well as regulated and dysregulated forms, is the bread and butter of most therapies. Emotion not only plays a central role in patient distress, but also in therapist understanding. For these reasons, I next explore how psychotherapy broadly and clinical intuition specifically implicate each of Panksepp's emotional and motivational circuits.

SEEKING*

The seeking instinct is the "granddaddy" of all other circuits (Panksepp, personal communication, July 2010) because it prompts us to explore our surroundings while experiencing pleasure and reward in the process. Enervated by dopamine, an excitatory transmitter and major source of arousal, the seeking circuit includes the ventral tegmental area and the nucleus accumbens as two major centers originating deep in the center of the brain (see Figure 3.6).

Although many patients feel "forced" into psychotherapy by a crisis, most psychotherapists directly tap into the seeking circuit by experiencing intrinsic rewards within the search for self-understanding and growth. During the heat of psychotherapy, both the memory and promise of inherent rewards can supply fuel and fortitude for our darkest moments. Within patients, I suspect that this circuit becomes co-opted during the transition from short-term, symptom-focused psychotherapy to open-ended, long-term psychotherapy, where more freedom exists to explore the psyche for its own sake.

Allan Schore (personal communication, April 2010) has speculated that whereas outer exploration of the physical and social environment rests on the sympathetic branch of the autonomic nervous system, inner paths of exploration may rely more on the parasympathetic branch. This may help

---

*Emotional circuits appear in capital letters at first mention, and in lower-case throughout the rest of the book.

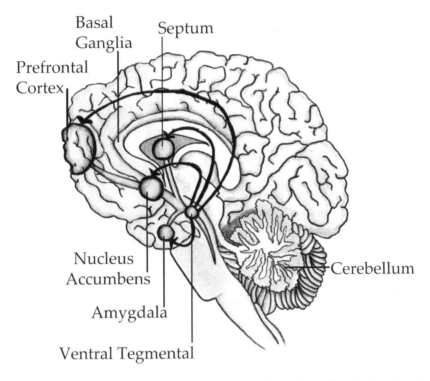

Basal Ganglia
Septum
Prefrontal Cortex
Nucleus Accumbens
Amygdala
Ventral Tegmental
Cerebellum

Figure 3.6. In response to carrying out vital functions, like finding food, shelter, and a mate, the seeking circuit (also called the reward circuit) provides feedback in the form of pleasurable sensations. Upon receiving and processing sensory information indicating a reward, the ventral tegmental area becomes activated. Information about how well basic needs are being met is then forwarded to various areas, including the nucleus accumbens, septum, amygdala, and prefrontal cortex, by using the neurotransmitter dopamine. The nucleus accumbens activates motor functions in the cerebellum and basal ganglia for a behavioral response, while the prefrontal cortex focuses attention in accordance. (Courtesy of the author.)

to explain the inherently self-soothing value of self-reflection, including the more formalized practice of mindfulness (Siegel, 2007, 2010). The seeking circuit, along with the care circuit, accounts for the clinician's broad interest, if not fascination, with people.

CARE

The care circuit constitutes the primary drive for parents to protect, care for, love, and nurture their babies. In many species of mammals, the care circuit extends to bonding with a particular mate to create a parental unit. The anthropologist Helen Fisher (1994) thought that, among humans across various cultures, romantic love drives people to attach to a single mate in order to coparent offspring, while lust drives people in the opposite direction to cheat with multiple partners in order to spread genetic seeds more widely.

Babies need to be touched, cuddled, doted on, worried over, gazed at, worshipped, sung to, meditated on, fantasized about, apologized to, and showered with every nuance of emotion. These emotional ingredients are as vital as air, food, and water in order for our children to grow up feeling internally safe and externally resilient. John Bowlby, a British psychiatrist and psychoanalyst, proved with his attachment theory (1969, 1973), that babies instinctively seek a secure emotional bond with their primary caregivers.

Bowlby personally knew the pain of early separation from his own mother. To ensure he would not become spoiled, Bowlby's mother met with him daily for only one hour over tea. When he turned 7, he was sent away to boarding school as was customary of the era. Bowlby struggled terribly, later stating, "I wouldn't send a dog away to boarding school at age seven" (Schwartz, 1999, p. 225). Bowlby emerged from these traumatic roots to retain empathy toward children's suffering throughout life. He passed his passion on to his son, Sir Richard Bowlby, who continues to champion his father's causes, in part through lobbying against the dangers of early daycare.

John Bowlby worked closely with ethologists, including Harry Harlow, an American colleague who studied the impact of maternal deprivation on monkeys. By rearing some rhesus monkeys with real mothers and comparing them to others raised with either wire or terrycloth inert versions, Harlow established the critical need for emotional care and companionship apart from physical needs (see Figure 3.7).

Harlow's research protocols were harsh and controversial. For example, they also included raising macaque monkeys in total isolation. Yet his work helped to spread empathy beyond the human realm by confirming that all young mammals seek proximity to sensitive, responsive adults as a secure base. Ironically, such methods would never pass ethical standards today, in part because they spawned the very animal rights movement that now prevents emotional and physical cruelty during experimentation.

Mary Ainsworth, another American colleague, extended Bowlby's work surrounding the mammalian care circuit to human toddlers. Ainsworth developed a research protocol named the Strange Situation Procedure (Ainsworth & Bowlby, 1965), which enabled her to observe and study stranger anxiety, separation distress, and reunion behavior. The protocol also allowed a more formal classification of different attachment styles. Ainsworth identified one form of secure and two forms of insecure attachment.

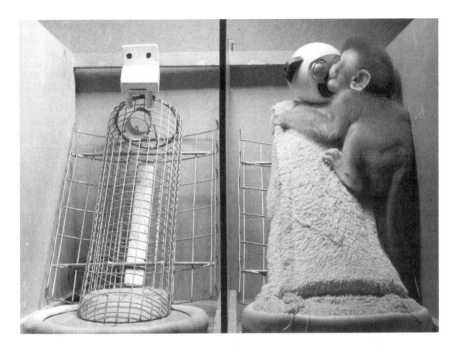

Figure 3.7. This infant monkey with mother surrogates made of wire and cloth was studied by Harry Harlow for research on maternal separation and deprivation. (Courtesy of Harlow Primate Laboratory, University of Wisconsin, Madison)

The securely attached baby, occupying roughly 65% of the population (Prior & Glaser, 2006), responds optimally to a mother's steady availability, emotional understanding, and full involvement. Feeling safe and secure, such a baby is free to openly explore the environment and play in his or her mother's presence. During the Strange Situation Procedure, although a baby is visibly upset when the mother leaves the room, while resisting the care of strangers, the baby is readily and quickly soothed back to a happy, relaxed state upon the mother's re-entry, returning quickly back to play.

The anxious, insecure child responds to a mother's inconsistent emotional availability that is offered according to the mother's terms, rather than dictated by her baby's needs. As a result, the mother is sometimes emotionally present and sometimes is not, leaving the baby worried about impending separation. Preoccupied and hypervigilant, with a continual need to keeps tabs on mom's whereabouts, a baby's freedom to play becomes obstructed. When placed in the Strange Situation Procedure, the baby becomes upset when the mother leaves but remains resentful and resistant to re-engagement when she returns.

The avoidant, insecure child responds to a mother's repeated dismissals and rejection of emotion. Initially this causes high distress and protestation. But as the mother continues to ignore her baby's bids for engagement, eventually the baby loses hope in the mother's emotional availability and demonstrates less play and interest in exploring the environment broadly. During the Strange Situation Procedure, avoidant babies are neither fazed by the mother's departure nor excited by her return. Nor do they mind the presence of a stranger. Their inclination is to fly solo instead, turning toward self-soothing and stimulation and away from relationships as a source for need satisfaction.

Mary Main is another colleague of Bowlby's who later added a more severe, disorganized category as a third type of insecure attachment (e.g., Main & Solomon, 1990). This category arises in response to a primary caretaker who is so abusive, erratic, or otherwise alarming as to short-circuit all of a baby's adaptive coping strategies. The baby is safe neither turning toward others nor turning toward itself, becoming incredibly confused instead, as if trying to approach and avoid the mother at the same time. These babies may hit themselves or cry during separation from the mother, yet they will avoid contact upon her return. Without effective means to meet their inner needs, their only choice is to shut down inside and dissociate from intolerable experiences and feelings.

As a developmental framework, attachment theory has proven unusually effective and predictive. Whereas securely attached children are likely to have good self-esteem and lasting relationships and will have bright, successful futures, insecurely attached children tend to encounter problems, often lasting into adulthood, with school, forming relationships, and developing emotional and even physical symptoms. Those with disorganized attachment are most vulnerable to future psychiatric and medical conditions (Mash & Barkley, 2003; Zeanah, 2009).

Within clinical research, there is some indication that securely attached therapists demonstrate the greatest clinical expertise (Eels, 2001). Whether these individuals begin life from a secure base or earn their security later through secondary attachment figures or from psychotherapy appears less significant. The capacity for secure attachment lends psychotherapists viable internal working models to guide intuitively driven empathic responses. The care circuit provides therapists with the neural wiring that makes empathy possible, along with the motivation to use it. Our bodies are driven by subcortical urges toward attuned responding; our minds are filled with the subjective experience of caring about the well-being of patients.

Given that parental love and affection constitute the hub of the care circuit, perhaps clinical intuition operates partly in service of loving our patients as if they were our children. A few clinical writers (e.g., Hirsch & Kessel, 1985; Lewis, Amini, & Lannon, 2000; Natterson, 2003; Shaw,

2003) speak of love during psychotherapy as a hidden but critical aspect of the healing stream. The capacity for therapists to love may be a nonspecific factor, which cross-cuts all modalities and theoretical orientations. Within the history of psychoanalysis, Freud placed the capacity to fall in love with one's therapist at the center of the transference dynamic. Love between patients and therapists proved a two-way street among some of our field's early luminaries. However, the impulse to act on romantic feelings and fantasies mirrors the incest taboo, with the destructive potential considered an abuse of power now protected by laws in most states prohibiting sex between therapists and patients. Still, if love is a key ingredient to healing, then as therapists it behooves us to separate out strands of lust from those of parental care within countertransference.

Empathy

The importance of love within psychotherapy is controversial and remains to be empirically determined. But the importance of empathy, which also derives from the care circuit, is not controversial. I can still remember a harrowing day during my graduate school training when I heard a woman screaming over and over to a fellow intern, "But you just don't understand! You don't understand!" If there is one ingredient that all therapists need in their tool boxes, it is the capacity to understand. The capacity to put ourselves in the shoes of our patients, both in an emotional as well as a cognitive sense, emanates from the same right-lateralized mammalian care circuit as intuition.

The capacity for empathy by necessity involves intuition partly by requiring parents to perceive and process novelty. Each baby is different. Each is endowed with a unique set of genes, personality predispositions, cultural milieu, family history, historical era, geographic location, and so on. What feels overwhelming for one baby might feel pleasurable to another. This incredible variation between children of all ages is precisely why parents need intuition to guide them while raising children. There is no parent manual that applies to all babies at all times. In order to be empathically attuned, parents must feel their way into their babies' inner worlds, quite literally starting with touch, smell, sight, sound, and full body involvement with all senses wide open.

When all goes well, by intuitively sensing babies' feelings, needs, motivations, and other inner states, parents (along with therapists) use instinctual faculties to serve the following functions:

- Down-regulate arousal of negative emotion, soothing baby's upset;
- Up-regulate arousal of positive emotion; stimulate and engage baby when he or she is calm, alert, and open for engagement;

- Help the baby to find the self through empathic attunement to the contours of changing inner needs and states;
- Process the baby's and parents' emotions to provide a safe container for the baby's self to flourish;
- Receive and extend invitations into intersubjective space, where mutual awareness of both people—their feelings, needs, and inner states—exists simultaneously; facilitating the relationship as it leads both into new territory, including new facets of self; and
- Use intersubjective space to color the baby's experience and scaffold an expansion into the larger physical and social world through exploration and play.

Clinical intuition mirrors parental intuition for each function above as illustrated by clinical examples in sections to come. Within psychotherapy, as during parenting, an attuned response does not involve fixed or preconceived ideas. Instead, empathy requires close, intuitively guided attention to moment-to-moment emotional shifts and fluctuations in energy and motivation. Such shifts are too tiny to list, much less to remember or plan around.

PLAY

Play is a separate motivational circuit that enjoys two chapters of its own. In this chapter I wish only to emphasize that, as with parents, the spirit of play blends seamlessly with the caring circuit. Meanwhile in children the spirit of play blends seamlessly with the developing self-system plus the child's capacity to orient and navigate in social space. These are serious functions, and play is no frivolous matter. I maintain that psychotherapy enjoys this same blend among caring, play, self-development, and social fluidity. A major purpose of this book is to elevate these areas of implicit understanding among parents into the explicit domain among psychotherapists.

RAGE

At first blush, therapists might reflexively recoil from the possibility that rage plays an important role within clinical intuition. But in clinical work, as in life, there is a time and place for every emotion. The therapeutic value of rage is illustrated by an amazingly raw and honest clinical vignette (Knox, 2010) where a psychoanalyst, stuck for month after month in an impasse with a nonresponsive patient, finally lost control of himself. The man blurted out, "I hate you, and I really hope you decide to leave therapy," to which his patient responded, "Thank god you have come back from the dead." This story, among many others, implicates the importance of bringing the whole self into the room with patients, which includes all of our emotional responses. Some therapists (e.g., Kaslow, Cooper, & Linsenberg, 1979; Miller et al., 1999; Rustin, 1970) place authenticity near the top, if not at the top, of the list of key therapist qualities.

Yet the power of rage, just like that of love, is a double-edged sword that needs careful wielding. Here is a counterexample from my own practice where unexpressed rage was enough to drive a patient from therapy. Bill had been recently hospitalized for a number of months due to a schizophrenic break. On his ward, he met, befriended, and fell in love for the first time with a fellow patient. This young lady was hospitalized to recover from a recent, serious suicide attempt. Although it was forbidden to act on romantic feelings in the hospital, after leaving, Bill began craving a physical relationship with this young woman. But, alas, she turned him down in service of retaining the friendship.

Here is the story that Bill told me in therapy one day, after the young woman yet again refused his advances. With her standing right in front of him and watching, Bill faked a suicide attempt. He pretended to swallow a fatal dose of pills. Then he followed this up several minutes later by swooning and falling to the ground. As I listened, I felt my body swell up with strong negative emotion—contempt, disgust, anger. At the time, I was less aware of my own lack of empathy for Bill and more trying to fathom his lack of empathy and the cruelty implied by the gesture. Intellectually I knew Bill was doing the best he could. Emotionally I could not stave off my visceral reaction. Although I said nothing, surely my feelings were written all over my face. Shortly afterward, the young man dropped out of treatment.

The psychoanalyst Harold Searles said the following on matters such as this:

> In the . . . core phase of the work with any one patient, each of the two participant's facial expressions "belong," in a sense, as much to the other as to oneself. In the work with a very ill patient, the therapist may find himself grimacing and having agonized (or other) facial expressions of a kind and degree that feel considerably foreign to him, and that are largely a response to dissociated feelings on the patient's part. (1984/1985, p. 60)

Searles had a schizophrenic mother. This must have acutely sensitized him to primitive expressions that cemented his deeply embodied, noninterpretive style, escalating his intuitive faculties well ahead of his day, especially when working with psychotic patients. Searles went on to state, "Only insofar as both participants can accept partial responsibility for such phenomena . . . can the patient's previously largely dissociated emotionality become more truly his own, and the therapist's face come to feel, once again, more fully his (the therapist's) own" (p. 60).

What a nice description of how rage can resonate in the intersubjective space between patient and therapist. As Allan Schore might put it, one amygdala picks up and reflects the dissociated emotion of another amygdala. Rapid face processing takes place at approximately 170 milliseconds, well beneath the threshold of consciousness (Dawson, Webb, & McPartland, 2005). The contempt that leaked through my body and onto my face felt much as Searles described—utterly alien. Not feeling like myself, I shocked myself while also hating how I felt. Unfortunately, the incident occurred far too soon into treatment; there simply was not enough relational glue to withstand the blow.

FEAR

Given that rage and fear are both energized by the same sympathetically driven, catecholaminergic channels, the two circuits often go hand in hand. Rage easily begets fear; fear in turn readily sparks rage; at the level of arousal, both relate to intense excitement. All this happens beneath the realm of awareness. Especially for people who experience their own vulnerability as dangerous, fear easily triggers rage, which feels safer. But these circuits also become coupled between people, as when one person's fear triggers another's rage. This may be one reason why victims of sexual and physical abuse sometimes seem to attract new abusers. Within the therapeutic community, clinical lore holds that fear often lurks at deeper, more unconscious levels within patients who are habitually enraged, while anger lurks at deeper, more unconscious levels within those who are habitually fearful.

In order to illustrate the role of the fear circuit during an intuitive moment with a patient, I here introduce the case of Macy. Macy originally sought psychotherapy because of violent tendencies toward her then boyfriend, accompanied by a strong desire to interrupt a long cycle of intergenerational violence.

The following exchange took place about a year into treatment.

"That stupid asshole!" exclaimed Macy about her boyfriend. "After a long day of work I come home to find him sitting on his ass in front of that stupid computer." Her voice began rising in tone, her volume getting louder. "I work my ass off while he sits on his to mess up the house."

"I can see how angry you were . . ." I replied.

Macy was too amped up to respond to my attempts at interactional regulation. Instinctively I modulated my voice by using a lower tone and slower pacing. But Macy interrupted with, "You're damned right! The laundry's in a pile on the floor. No dinner on the table. The guy just sits there like a fucking idiot. He isn't even using the computer for work. Do you know what he was doing? That asshole was playing games. Just like a stupid child. That's what he looked like sitting there—like a stupid child."

"You really found it hard to respect him," I squeezed in.

"Who could respect that guy?" Macy shot back, her rage continuing to escalate until she was shouting at the top of her lungs, spit spraying, her arms wildly gesticulating as she continued on. "He doesn't deserve respect. He's not even a man. He's just pathetic. He's a wimp. He wouldn't even look at me in the eye. He was such a pussy, cowering like he was scared of me."

"But you are scary!" I replied softly.

Macy stopped in her tracks, her voice tone now lower and slower. "What did you say?"

I repeated, "I said you are scary. You scared me when you got riled up just now—simply by telling me what happened. I can imagine how frightened your boyfriend must have felt actually being there with you."

Macy looked puzzled. "Are you saying that I scare you? That's hard to believe."

"Why?"

"Because you look so calm. You always look like you have everything under control."

"That's not how I always feel. While you were shouting a moment ago, I could feel my heart thumping. My breath was coming quick. The more worked up you got, the more I was quivering inside."

Macy retained that puzzled look on her face, "But what are you afraid of? Do you think I would hurt you?"

"No, not physically. I trust you that way. I was just afraid. Period. I don't know. The more out of control you looked, the more out of control I started to feel."

This was not an intervention I had planned. It was an intuitive moment. After working with Macy for more than a year, I spontaneously took the risk of disclosing my fear in reaction to her display of rage. It could have backfired. Macy could have turned her rage onto me in that moment. But she did not, and this proved a pivotal moment.

Previously Macy intellectually understood that she contributed to her relationship problems, but she did not really understand how. She automatically assumed that her boyfriend was to blame whenever she flew off the handle. After all, he was triggering her rage, was he not? He should have known better. Macy had a blind spot. She had a deficit in empathy that she could not see. During this pivotal therapy moment, Macy both understood and felt compassion for my fear of her. In turn, this stimulated greater respect and empathy for similar reactions within her boyfriend.

Recent evidence shows that children and adolescents are less sensitive to the perception of fear and anger on the faces of others, because their neural underpinnings are not yet fully developed (Thomas, DeBellis, Graham, & LaBar, 1997). This may have been part of the story for Macy, who instead interpreted her boyfriend's facial and postural cues in emasculating and humiliating ways. While our clinical moment of meeting did not stop Macy from having abusive tirades, it did help to slow down their frequency and severity. And on those occasions when Macy did lose control of her temper, she no longer automatically assumed that her boyfriend was at fault or that he deserved her abuse.

Here is how I see what happened. My willingness to share my vulnerability in the context of a strong bond and mutual respect activated Macy's care circuit along with her protective instincts toward me. Throughout our psychotherapy sessions, Macy continually expressed gratitude for how protected and nurtured she felt by me. Unlike with Bill, the patient who faked the suicide attempt, my own rage and contempt were not an issue. Perhaps because I saw how hard Macy was trying, I never felt inclined to shame or humiliate her for losing self-control. Similarly I never threatened to abandon Macy as a patient, despite her continual fears of "being fired" in retribution for these lapses.

This moment of meeting bestowed upon Macy the first taste of expanded empathy, first for me and then for her boyfriend, who eventually became her husband. From a place of caring, Macy could take in the vulnerability of my perspective and honor it. The final vignette of this chapter reveals how Macy eventually extended her capacity for empathy still farther, toward her own infant.

PANIC

Panksepp (1998) identified the panic circuit as being central to the attachment system. Babies and young children panic at separation because their lives depend on the close, attuned presence of critical caregivers in a literal and concrete way. The panic of separation plus the grief of loss represent the survival-oriented flip side of inborn capacities to bond and love. A baby's cry is the prototypical expression of the panic of separation. In turn, within parents there exist specialized areas of their limbic circuitry that attend preferentially to cries as well as to laughs (Swain, in press). Along with the amygdala, this circuitry also includes the anterior cingulate cortex, specialized to perceive physical and emotional pain, and the insula, which monitors our own body states plus the bodies of others. From the start and throughout development, the human cry is so significant and nuanced that Judith Kay Nelson (2005) has written a whole book about its variations. Whether babies feel hungry, tired, or physically uncomfortable, newborns do not cry primarily out of need; they cry because they are wired to communicate their needs to critical caregivers. The capacity of caregivers to decode the meaning of the cry and respond in turn is a major source of self-agency for the infant within early development (Knox, 2010).

Returning to the interspecies example of Mila and the diver, recall that it was at the point that the diver panicked that Mila came to the rescue. It is likely that Mila's amygdala picked up on Yun's distress. Whales and humans both have especially large and well-developed amygdaloid systems (Perrin, Würsig, & Thewissin, 2008). During evolution, this system arose in tandem with the olfactory bulb (smell) and possibly the auditory system (hearing). From an evolutionary perspective, both smell and hearing are critical senses for predators and prey alike to detect one another.

Mila's story also underscores deep neural connections between the panic circuit and primitive dangers of suffocation. Consider this: The baby's first act of separation from a mother comes literally when taking his or her first breath. Severed from the safety of the umbilical cord, if the baby does not breathe, he or she will die. There is a connection between panic and lack of oxygen that sheds light on why panic so easily breeds more panic. The more we panic, the more rapidly and shallowly we breathe, depriving us of oxygen, which in turn stimulates more panic. During panic, higher cortical centers that use more oxygen get deprived of oxygen first. Someone can run around like a chicken without its head partly because the subcortical limbic areas mature and become fully operational under anaerobic conditions, without the benefit of oxygen, within the womb. Finally this connection between panic and suffocation may shed light on why tidal waves appear as recurrent, archetypal dream images that symbolize separation distress, as illustrated by Sabina's clinical vignette in the last chapter.

NEUROBIOLOGY OF MIND READING

The ability to feel our way into the minds, bodies, and lives of others derives from nurturance and social bonding instincts wired deep within the brain and body. As babies we have immature nervous systems that render us helpless, open, vulnerable, and responsive to the input of others, for good and for bad. As parents we do our best to love and nurture our young, not just in body but also in mind and heart, by attending to their feelings, needs, motives, fantasies, and other inner states. This open circuitry lends additional flexibility, learning, and complexity to the human repertoire, permitting us to reach new heights of imagination, language, society, and culture.

The neural wiring of parent/child relatedness operates as a two-way street. Parents instinctually read the states, needs, and motives of infants, while from day one babies respond to implicit communications from parents. If all proceeds smoothly, there is mutuality. As a baby's needs get met, the baby comes to know the contours of the self through sensing the contours of others. Both people are emotionally present; both are relationally melded. Each feels the self reach new places in the presence of the other. As therapists, we have the capacity to set aside agendas, to let go of "doing to" in order to "be with," and this allows a similar kind of attunement to minute-to-minute fluctuations. Much like the early exploration between a mother and baby, the mutual state locating the self-within-other and other-within-self continually yields novel experiences, providing rich opportunities for intuitive responding from both sides of the couch.

Within a large body of research on empathy, mind reading is considered the ability to attribute mental states to other people, in order to understand, explain, or predict their behavior (Goldman, 2008; Kalbe et al., 2010). What do others feel? What do they believe? What drives their behavior? What do they intend? Some researchers call this capacity to put ourselves in the shoes of another theory of mind; others call it mentalizing (e.g., Fonagy, Gergely, Jurist, & Target, 2004). In the developmental literature, it is often called perspective taking (e.g., Burns & Brainerd, 1979). Whatever name we choose for this ability, these capacities for empathy are foundational to the operation of clinical intuition (see Figure 3.8).

Mind reading is most often identified as a right-brain function, stemming from openness of the right hemisphere to the interconnectedness of things, its interest in others as individuals, plus concern with how we relate to them:

> If I imagine myself in pain, I use both hemispheres, but your pain is in my right hemisphere. The same neurons in the right anterior cingulate cortex, an area known to be associated with the appreciation of pain, show activity whether we ourselves are hurt or we witness someone else undergoing a similar painful experience. . . . When we put ourselves in others' shoes, we are using the right inferior parietal lobe, and the right lateral prefrontal cortex, which is involved in inhibiting the automatic tendency to espouse one's own point of view. In circumstances of right-hemisphere activation, subjects are more favourably disposed towards others and more readily convinced by arguments in favour of positions that they have not previously supported. (McGilchrist, 2009, p. 57)

McGilchrist described how the ability to mind read first evolved in our primate ancestors along with self-recognition and self-awareness, which are closely linked skills. Within humans, the precursors to mind reading emerge around the ages of 12 to 18 months, when the frontal lobes begin to mature. The skill develops more fully around the age of 4 as indicated by the classic research paradigm for identifying mind reading. Children are shown two puppets, Stella and Sue, who together are playing with a marble. When the dolls finish playing, they put the marble away in a box and leave the room. In a short while, Stella returns alone. She takes out the marble and plays with it for a little while. Then she puts it away inside a different box before leaving the room once again. Here is the critical question: When Sue returns, where she will look for the marble? Children that lack a theory of mind, along with autistic individuals, select the second box where they know the marble actually will be. Those with theory of mind choose instead the box where Sue first saw the marble to be placed.

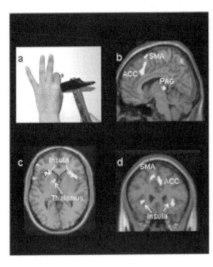
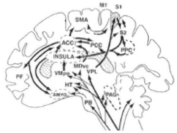

The pain matrix involves a complex network of brain structures and pathways containing both serial and parallel connections.

→ The primary (S1) and secondary (S2) sensory cortices are involved in the sensory-discriminative dimension of pain, e.g., the bodily location, intensity, and duration of the noxious stimuli.

→ The ACC and anterior insula subserve the affective-motivational component, i.e., the evaluation of subjective discomfort in the context of painful or aversive stimuli.

Figure 3.8. It is no coincidence that we use the same word—"pain"—for the physical hurt of our bodies and the social hurt of exclusion or poor treatment by others. The same underlying brain pathways are involved. Furthermore, the neural network for processing our own pain overlaps greatly with that for perceiving others in distress. To perceive pain in others recruits brain areas primarily involved in affective and motivational processing (the anterior cingulate cortex [ACC], insula), plus the somatosensory cortex and periaqueductal gray (PAG). The anterior insula helps with sensory coding, body state assessment, autonomic regulations, and assigning emotional valence to sensory events. The cingulate cortex helps with affect regulation, including avoidant and defensive responses to pain. (Courtesy of Jean Decety)

The protocol above clearly is a cognitive test of empathy. One way of discerning this is because the stakes are really low here. No one is suffering; it does not really matter whether anyone gets the whereabouts of the marble wrong. The emotional capacity for empathy is all about suffering. On the one hand, just as animals are instinctively attuned to their masters' distress, so are babies. Over the past 10 years much research has been amassed on empathy in babies and toddlers (see Decety & Ickes, 2009). For example, very young children have been shown to tell the difference between books purposely thrown down and those dropped in the same way out of frustration. These babies do not respond in the former case but rush in to help in the latter case.

Mind reading involves complex neural circuitry, including the right medial prefrontal cortex (mPFC), superior temporal sulcus region, temporal pole, and amygdala (e.g., Adolphs, 2003; Siegel & Varley, 2002). Recent evidence (Hynes, Baird, & Grafton, 2006; Kalbe et al, 2010) suggests two distinct, dissociable aspects for perspective taking: One is cognitive, and the other is affective. Each possesses distinct neural circuitry within the right prefrontal cortex. The ventromedial prefrontal cortex (VMPFC) appears to be the seat of affective dimensions of empathy, while the dorsolateral prefrontal cortex (DLPFC) appears to house cognitive aspects (see Figure 3.9).

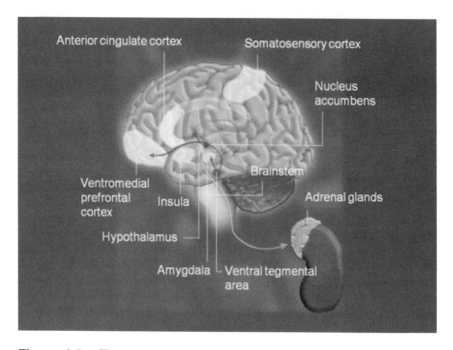

Figure 3.9. The general mammalian neural circuitry of reward and social attachment and the brain pathways of empathy enable humans to care for and about others. A wide range of underlying brain areas participates within the cortex, limbic system, midbrain, and brainstem. The arousal regulating the autonomic nervous system, HPA axis, and endocrine system also contributes to empathy by helping to regulate arousal, bodily states, emotion, and reactivity. High-level cognitive abilities of executive function, language, and mentalizing get layered atop phylogenetically older social and emotional capacities. These evolutionarily newer aspects of information processing expand the potential range of responses. They also lend flexibility for helping others outside of the immediate kin, social group, or even species. (Courtesy of Jean Decety)

These two dimensions might reflect different underlying processes at work during perspective taking. Simulation theory suggests that we understand other people's inner worlds by mimicking their internal states as we slip into their shoes. The burgeoning study of mirror neurons in the premotor frontal cortex, which fire whenever we or someone else conducts an action such as reaching for a handshake, is also part of simulating the inner worlds of others. Simulation theory reflects the emotional aspect of empathy.

"Theory theory" suggests a more rational process by which we model the inner worlds of others through manipulating knowledge systems that exist apart from our own mental states. Theory theory reflects the cognitive aspect of perspective taking. Some researchers (Shamay-Tsoory, Tomer, Berger, Goldsher, & Aharon-Peretz, 2005) suggested a two-step process by which the automatic, quick-acting affective dimension of empathy serves as the foundation for later cognitive, decision-making processes that pose more metabolic and cognitive demands on inner resources. This is consistent with the developmental sequence whereby the amygdala and limbic portion of the VMPFC matures earlier than the nonlimbic DLPFC.

As clinicians, we clearly utilize both emotional and cognitive aspects of empathy. In fact, sensing when to switch between purely emotional and more cognitive dimensions is a central aspect of clinical intuition. At times it is important to bask together with our patients in mutual feeling states. At other times we need to figure out the mind of the other in order to become oriented within a clinical moment. This especially holds when cognitive understanding facilitates affective experience by providing a safe context.

Throughout my clinical work with Macy, helping her to understand how the brain works has served as a nonjudgmental, nonshaming way to process violent residues of early trauma. Yet the shift from affective sharing through "being with" to more cognitive understanding can interrupt the flow of experience, especially if we switch gears too quickly. To make these choices, right-brain intuition is much more effective than left-brain rationality in guiding the timing. From the start, humans are wired to flesh out the inner worlds of each other, except where previous trauma or neurological problems stand in the way of accessing these faculties. The ability to take the perspective of another, both emotionally and cognitively, lies at the heart of a baby's neural development, parental instincts, and clinical intuition. I close this chapter with one more vignette where all three facets merge.

THE BIRTH OF INTERSUBJECTIVITY

Macy sought psychotherapy right about the time her boyfriend proposed. Macy knew she wanted children, and, given her proclivities toward violence, Macy wanted to prevent the extension of such trauma into yet another generation. In a long line of abuse begetting further abuse, Macy was the first and only person in her family to try the route of therapy. In fact she pursued psychotherapy against the advice of all relatives.

The more Macy calmed down and trusted me, the more she confronted her own need to control others through domination and humiliation. After being married for about a year, Macy became pregnant and then delivered a healthy baby girl. Macy was enraptured. She could hardly believe what a beautiful creature she and her husband had produced. She felt so much love, which she expressed by working hard to figure out just what the baby needed. What did that cry mean? Was this a howl of hunger? Perhaps the diaper was dirty? Was there too much spice in the breast milk? Macy prided herself on attending to these details to counter her own mother's neglect and abuse.

In the early months before she returned to work, Macy enjoyed bringing the baby to therapy and watching me dote. She relished seeing the baby receive comfort in my arms, as we sat and talked about the stresses and strains of her sleepless nights. I noticed my own relief at how naturally Macy took to motherhood and at how easily her baby melted into my arms. I recall my own rush of tenderness one session when I recognized that I was simultaneously soothing baby and mother while supplying something so lacking in Macy's own childhood.

One day when the baby was about 4 months old, Macy walked into therapy wheeling the carriage. The baby was wide awake, with her eyes riveted on her mom's face.

Macy commented casually, "She seems fascinated with your door frame."

"I don't think so," I responded. "I think she's looking at you."

"Nah," Macy shot back, "doesn't seem likely."

"You can't see that she's mesmerized by your face?"

"In your imagination," Macy quipped.

We went back and forth on this a couple more times. My inner alarm slowly started ringing. I realized with horror that Macy literally could not see her baby looking at her. As we talked more, I also realized Macy could not perceive her baby's smiles in response to what the baby saw.

As had become our custom, I eagerly scooped Macy's baby in my arms. But today, rather than settle the baby in so that I could give Macy my full attention, I did something different. I started gazing intently at the baby, bobbing my head around and grinning like a maniac. I began speaking in high-pitched melodic tones, often called "motherese," my pitch getting more and more feverish as I proceeded. Suddenly I nuzzled my head into the baby's soft belly, twisting my face around, sputtering loudly. Then just as suddenly I pulled my head away again so I could observe the baby's reaction. I did this over and over. Slowly the baby started to smile. Then she started to laugh. Her low-pitched gurgle dribbled into higher pitches.

Eventually the baby was emitting a full-bodied giggle in response to my own very high arousal states.

Macy sat in disbelief, with her mouth half open. She had never seen anything like this. She had not heard her baby giggle before. I looked up. Macy and I started to laugh. In another precious moment, Macy, I, and the baby were all ecstatic. As we settled in from this drunken joy, Macy and I reflected on what had just happened.

Until that moment, Macy had rather mechanically considered her baby little more than an eating, pooping, sleeping "blob." It had not crossed Macy's mind that at such a tender age her baby was capable of relating with her. Macy had carefully and lovingly done things for and around her daughter. But only at this point did Macy realize that her daughter also needed to be joined emotionally. In particular the baby needed to be looked at, with her affective states responded to. Suddenly Macy understood the source of her baby's recent restlessness—the fidgeting Macy had not been able to decipher as the baby made frantic bids for mom's attention.

A moment later, it occurred to me that when Macy walked into my office and was unable to receive her baby's eyes, this stemmed from Macy not being given the gift of her own mother's gaze. Macy's mother had carried on the family tradition of discriminating against little girls. Macy's mother was herself the victim of early abuse when her own mother, Macy's grandmother, had tried to kill her with bare hands upon learning she had delivered a baby girl and not a boy. I sensed that Macy's implicit working model held no early memory of her own mother's loving look.

Intuitively, this resonated for us both. There is no way to prove this, but the possibility accorded with later observations of Macy's mother in interactions with Macy's baby. Macy perceived no instinctive capacity to respond at all. Instead her mother either ignored the baby's emotions or initiated with her own theories. It is little wonder that Macy could not imagine seeking comfort from her own mother. Macy was blocked from feeling her own body's instinct toward that kind of engagement through an attachment bid. This point was brought home every time Macy observed how natural and instinctive such bids were within her own baby.

This session proved a pivotal point for Macy in relation to her baby. For me, the whole experience was an arc of joy rare in life, much less within psychotherapy. This precious moment, intuitively wrought, represented the "birth of intersubjectivity" between us all. Because Macy trusted and aligned with me so completely, she could borrow my eyes in order to see what I was seeing in her baby. Watching my capacity for empathy and relatedness expanded Macy's capacities naturally. Her baby's presence expanded from being a blob to a real person before her very eyes. It was a privilege to watch how the fruits of my clinical intuition further unlocked the inborn capacities of Macy's maternal intuition.

WRAP-UP

The topic of clinical intuition is tricky business. It is a phenomenon you recognize when you are in it but struggle to express. The concept is inherently vague and difficult to pin down apart from lived moments. Surely this is one reason why clinical intuition has received so little attention in outcome research. Yet as I have already mentioned, this is a topic so near and dear to us all as to constitute the proverbial air without which our therapeutic relationships might easily suffocate.

In this chapter, I shed light on the implicit, nonconscious, nonverbal origins of clinical intuition within the social emotions, motivations, and attachment circuits we share with mammals that nurture their young. These circuits prompt us to care for vulnerable others, including our patients. These circuits enable us to resonate with people's emotions and predicaments. They are the means through which we feel our way into the condition of patients' bodies, the suffering of their hearts, and the content of their minds. These circuits of empathy lend us what Reik (1983) called a third ear with which to listen and an inner eye with which to see a path to healing.

I offered a clinical case about the care circuit where early trauma interfered with a patient's capacity to empathize. Clinical intuition prompted me to take an emotional risk that proved worthwhile. A later vignette from the same patient revealed how her expanded capacity for empathy helped to birth intersubjectivity with her baby. By borrowing my eyes, she was able to transform her 4-month-old from a mere blob to an emotional being with needs to be seen and feel felt, as Daniel Siegel would say, just like herself. The first vignette I told was a tale of rage and fear, and the second, of excitement and joy. I ended with a breakthrough that involved positive emotion and intense arousal.

In order to sensitize yourself to your own empathic style of exhibiting care for others, it is useful to consider the following questions:

- What brings you flow with patients? How can you use your knowledge to increase your flow states?
- What is your implicit family mandate to go into this profession? What family dynamics contributed to your interest (e.g., rescuing sick others, being someone's sounding board)?
- How do your own dynamics leave you vulnerable in a countertransferential sense? What kinds of enactments are you most susceptible to fall into?
- Which of the different "flavors" of not-knowing most challenges your capacity for empathy—the ambiguity of too little information or the paradox of too much information that may be contradictory?

- When feeling anxious, some people dive into action and solution-seeking while others distract from discomfort and still others become paralyzed. What happens to you when you are challenged in this way?
- Which of the two aspects of empathy is your stronger suit—the emotional dimension of feeling other people's pain and emotional states, or the cognitive dimension of understanding their situations? What vulnerabilities as a clinician surround these leanings?

In the next chapter, we will examine the importance of the play circuit for psychotherapy.

CHAPTER 4

Play

Necessity may be the mother of invention, but play is certainly the father.

—Roger von Oech

Die Thiere spielen nicht, weil sie jung sind, sondern sie haben eine Jugend, weil sie spielen müssen." (The animals do not play because they are young, but they are young because they must play.)

—Karl Groos

AFTER BRAIN PLASTICITY, THE NEXT great development in the evolution of human knowledge was curiosity. Instead of merely responding to the press of innate survival needs, as reptiles do, mammals became, through play, proactive, adventurous, and inquisitive. Spencer (1873) viewed play as frivolous, a mere "aimless expenditure of exuberant energy" in children and young animals, while more contemporary developmental psychologists like Piaget (1962) regarded play as purposeful and even essential to human development. From a developmental perspective, the focus on play used to be as static, imitative depiction, reflecting society as it currently exists. The contemporary perspective has shifted to a more dynamic lens, viewing play's creative potential to transform both the individual and society at large (Linder, Roos, & Victor 2001).

In fact, the subject of play has been elevated to the point where an entire journal, the *American Journal of Play*, is now devoted to play's multidisciplinary exploration. The Strong National Museum of Play has also arisen in Rochester, New York (see Figure 4.1), as a hands-on approach to multifaceted aspects of play for children and families.

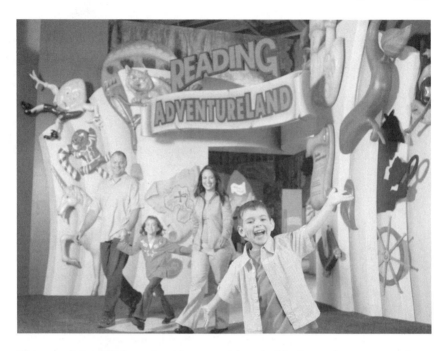

Figure 4.1. While play is considered frivolous by many, from evolutionary and developmental perspectives, it is central to mammalian and human development, encouraging learning, creativity, and discovery. Play affords us a safe context to move joyfully while internalizing culture and establishing identity. From the point of view of brain development, play is key to neural flexibility and plasticity. To honor the centrality of play to what makes us human, the Strong National Museum of Play, was founded in Rochester, New York, as the only collection-based museum in the world dedicated solely to this topic. (Courtesy of the Strong National Museum of Play)

Across all descriptive levels, neurobiological, psychological, sociological, and anthropological investigations have identified a host of affective, cognitive, social, and motor capacities that accompany children's play (for a summary, see Marks-Tarlow, 2010).

These include the following:

- Brain growth;
- Self-regulation of behavior and emotions;
- Development of imagination and symbolic representation;
- Meaning making;
- Development of language and narrative;
- Meta-communication (communication about communication);

- Creativity and divergent thinking;
- Self-transformation;
- Social competence;
- Gender identification;
- Community membership; and
- Cultural awareness and creation.

In this chapter, I review the role of play within psychotherapy. This is not to be confused with play therapy, a more formal usage that is especially popular with young children, or play from a Jungian perspective, which encourages the use of the sandtray with adults. Instead, I refer to the informal use of play during psychotherapy as it is orchestrated intuitively. Whether or not we are conscious of using it, because play is a major source for implicit learning within the social domain, I propose it as a nonspecific factor to therapeutic effectiveness that cross-cuts all modalities. Further, I suggest that play bears an important relationship to creativity, especially as it exists *in the intersubjective space between the therapist and patient.*

Sometimes clinicians sense the instinct to play coming to the fore, as when we consciously search for new possibilities with a lighthearted spirit or when we coconstruct safe experiments with patients to try at home or in the room. But more often play emerges implicitly, that is, automatically, in bottom-up fashion, as a primary tool of clinical intuition. In order to demonstrate how play arises spontaneously and intersubjectively, I begin with a clinical example. From there, I move on to the neurobiology of play and examine its emergence in the mammalian brain and its developmental role. In particular, I highlight the importance of play for increasing affect tolerance, offering behavioral flexibility, expanding positive emotion, creating intrinsic motivation, and broadening social skills and competencies.

EMOTIONAL RESILIENCE THROUGH PLAY

The red light goes on to signal a patient's presence. I check the clock. At precisely 3 P.M. I open the door to my waiting room. In walks Sylvia, a stunning young woman in her mid-twenties, sporting curly red hair, bohemian clothes, and work boots so old they are held together with duct tape. Sylvia greets me with a little wave and a sheepish smile as she slips past. I follow her into my office, remembering at the last minute to grab the watch off my desk. As I stand there waiting, watch in hand, Sylvia slowly surveys the room. Then she walks toward the couch and swivels in a semicircle on her heels. She goes over to the ottoman, picks it up, and sets it down between the couch and chair. Then Sylvia lowers herself onto it as if straddling a horse. I respond by walking to my desk, laying down my watch, then moving to my chair, which I turn to face Sylvia directly. I sit down. The session begins.

Before reading on, please take this opportunity to guess what just happened and why. What was this ritual all about? What made Sylvia survey the room? Why did I pick up the watch and then return it to my desk? Why did Sylvia move the ottoman? Take a couple of minutes to play with the scenario and see how many plausible or not-so-plausible speculations you can brainstorm. When ready, read on for some clinical background.

Sylvia came from a high-functioning, upper-middle-class family as the second youngest of four siblings, all close to one another and to parents who conscientiously cultivated a tight family unit. Unlike Sylvia's siblings, who grew up with only minor hiccups along the way, Sylvia was the anomaly of the family. She was different from the start—more emotional, unpredictable, rebellious, and untamed. While brilliant and witty, she struggled in high school and dropped out of college in the first semester. In 12th grade, Sylvia suffered a "nervous breakdown" that took the form of an existential crisis over the meaning of love. Sylvia's self-doubt and philosophical queries literally knocked her off her feet, rattling her world so completely that she became functionally paralyzed.

Sylvia's parents were stunned. They cared deeply about their daughter and only wanted what was best for her. But the more upset they became at Sylvia's condition and the more they tried to cater to their daughter's needs, the more anguished the young woman became. After being bedridden for months, Sylvia was eventually put on a cocktail of drugs. When she emerged from the bedroom, everyone crossed their fingers and hoped for the best. Yet no one still had a clue what was going on—Sylvia included.

Sylvia made her way from the small midwestern town where she grew up to Southern California, where she found her way to me. From the start, the wild rebellious child in me connected with this young woman. My own father was a *puer aeternus* (eternal child) and I, as mentioned previously, was his confidante. My father's primary implicit message was to enjoy life to the fullest and never get trapped—not in a fixed job, not in a confining marriage, and especially not in meaningless convention. Intuitively I "got" Sylvia from the start. I understood her desire to break the mold, her leanings toward outlandish idealism, her worship of funny people, her desperation to be creative no matter who gets alienated, and her simultaneous dread of alienating anyone at all, even the busboy.

From Sylvia's perspective, I instantly served as a fabulous role model as the only adult she knew who felt free, loved her work, wore flowing clothes, moved with a light step, and roared with raucous laughter. From the start, Sylvia wanted my admiration and easily stole the gleam in my eye. Every time I looked at this young woman, I saw a soiled shiny gem wildly sputtering with potential. When Sylvia said something smart, I responded in kind. When she curled into a ball, I quietly witnessed. When she sank toward the floor, my head tilted sideways. When she said something funny, I guffawed.

Little did I suspect that the fact that I laughed was a litmus test of my worth as a therapist. Sylvia had tried therapy once before. Her previous therapist sat stiffly in the chair, receiving the young woman's every utterance in a solemn manner. Instead of trusting Sylvia's impulse to break out of and temper her pain with wit, this therapist interpreted Sylvia's use of humor as a defense. This was not my gut reaction. For I could feel the humor spreading between us like thick honey, gluing us together to soothe Sylvia's isolation and rough edges.

In counterpoint to these bursts of wit in my office, in general Sylvia was bound so tightly she could hardly breathe. I suggested that she try yoga to relax and ground herself more fully within her physical body. Meanwhile, every time Sylvia came for her twice-weekly sessions, I tried to ensure that she felt free. Sylvia could talk about anything without my judgment—fear of overwhelming others, sex as reassurance, love of brilliant shock jocks, envy for comics who wear vulnerability like a badge. Sometimes Sylvia focused on big issues, other times on tiny details. Every session had an edge of play, an element of naughtiness. No matter what topic she landed on, I eagerly followed. Yet no matter what she said, I tended to find deep meaning, sometimes on and sometimes under the surface. Meanwhile, Sylvia was all over the map emotionally.

Dear reader, here is a second opportunity to guess what was taking place at the beginning of the session before reading on. . . .

To me, each patient is unique. No matter how many anxious people I see, no two look alike. Every patient is perfect, having found the perfect adaptation for emotional, social, and physical challenges faced. Every patient is clever, sometimes too clever for his or her own good, using cleverness to evade self-awareness. Finally, each patient offers up a mystery: Where is the pain? What are the symptoms? How do these adaptations make sense in light of current circumstances and previous history? What is the key to change, healing, and growth? Through the play of intuition, I sleuth about in search of clues to these initial questions, inviting my patients to be cosleuths along the way.

Sylvia presented a special kind of mystery; she had such severe symptoms, yet she came from such a loving, intact family with no obvious stressors. Here is what I pieced together developmentally. Unlike her siblings, Sylvia was a difficult baby. Her emotions were so big her parents could not attend to them. Mom became disheartened at her baby's wails and tended to pass Sylvia to Dad. Dad tolerated the narcissistic blow of the baby's inconsolability better, but eventually, when none of his tricks worked, both parents felt scared and overwhelmed. What were they doing wrong? Was there something really wrong with Sylvia? Why *couldn't they make* their baby feel better?

As Sylvia grew, rather than using the steady eye of her parents to become grounded inside her own body and comfortable with her range of emotions, Sylvia was far too aware of her mother's feelings of being over-whelmed and her dad's vulnerabilities. Sylvia blamed herself. She was much too much for everybody and certainly too much for herself. She could not stand the intensity of what she felt, especially her perceived impact on others, and she could not imagine feeling differently. The pressure was too much. The intense highs and lows of her internal experience were so overwhelming that she compensated by flattening her external world. At a certain point Sylvia concluded that if you stay very low and rest very still on the ground, there is nowhere else to fall.

Enter psychotherapy, as informed by Winnicott's sensibilities:

> Psychotherapy takes place in the overlap of two areas of playing, that of the patient and that of the therapist. Psychotherapy has to do with two people playing together. The corollary of this is that where playing is not possible then the work done by the therapist is directed towards bringing the patient from a state of not being able to play into a state of being able to play. (1971, p. 44)

From the start I intuited play as a path to healing for Sylvia. Everything had become too scary. The stakes were too high. Every social encounter was too serious. The risks were not worth taking. Even if Sylvia succeeded one minute, everything could change the next. Without a relational frame to contain her high arousal and variability, Sylvia could not inhabit her own nature fully. Implicitly I sensed that Sylvia was out of sync with her own playful nature as being deeply wired into her character. She needed another playmate, one with a tolerance for great intensity. Voilà—our good-enough fit.

Within months of beginning psychotherapy, Sylvia took to yoga. She slowly weaned herself off all medication under the guidance of a psychiatrist. Within a year Sylvia had enrolled in a community college. Within 2 years she transferred with very high grades to a prestigious 4-year university. Within 3 years she took stabs at creative writing she had dreamed about before, but could not discipline herself to dare.

Last chance to guess at the opening shenanigans in my office . . .

I have been giving you lots of background about Sylvia to illustrate how play was vital to her healing process. As we came to know one another, Sylvia and I had developed a unique nonverbal ritual. At the beginning of each session, I made no assumptions about where and how Sylvia would sit. She was free to arrange my furniture in any way she wished; I responded accordingly. The one exception was my chair, which I retained the right to sit in, though even that convention was eventually tossed. Sometimes Sylvia landed on the couch, other times on the matching chair to mine. Occasionally she would sprawl out on the floor or would wind up at some odd angle "in the space between" various pieces of furniture. This was how she arranged the ottoman as described earlier. It was all part of the play between us. Each session, as Sylvia entered my office I would grab my watch from the desk in case I wound up facing away from the clock. I would then either put it on or return the watch to my desk if I could see the clock (I hate wearing watches if I do not have to).

At times there was consistency to Sylvia's choices. The couch started off representing vulnerability, and the chair was self-support. Then the couch morphed into authenticity while the chair represented counterdependency. Part of the rules of our implicitly emerging game included flexibility for the rules to change along with Sylvia's inner world. In contrast to the inescapable quicksand of her psyche, the physical or intersubjective space of my office (see Figure 4.2) became a place of greater lightness and fluidity.

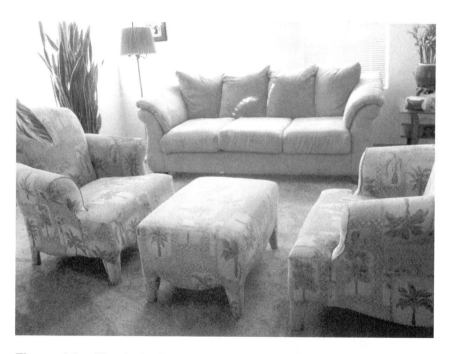

Figure 4.2. The feel of a psychotherapy office tells much about the character of the therapist. Traditional psychoanalytic offices were dark, at least stereotypically so—a dark brown leather couch, dark wood desks and even floors, and pulled shades to facilitate inner journeys. As the reader can see in this picture, my office is quite light, both in colors and there is lots of sunlight streaming through the windows. Perhaps there is a geographical component. After all, I do live in sunny Southern California. Beyond that, there is a metaphorical component to the lightness, for I believe my greatest strengths as a therapist involve helping others to lighten their loads. (Courtesy of the author)

From a developmental perspective, the Russian psychologist Lev Vygotsky (1978) viewed play as taking place within a zone of proximal development. This represents the cutting edge, the place of safety to try out new ways of being and doing. During play is when new mastery is likely; indeed, during play, children demonstrate new cognitive, emotional, social, and behavioral abilities well before they do so in nonplay contexts (Marks-Tarlow, 2010). This certainly held true for Sylvia. The flexible arrangement of furniture proved an outer embodiment of our relationship, which helped to grease inner wheels. Over time Sylvia came to feel more powerful while embracing a more flexible self-image.

By arranging the room according to spontaneous, immediate whim and by watching me adjust accordingly, Sylvia got a taste of self-agency at its most primitive level. Jean Knox (2010) wrote that the infant's first act of agency is the capacity to move her parents in accordance with her inner need. Developmentally, the infant comes into this world too helpless and dependent to affect anything beyond his or her own body directly. The first spark of self-agency consists in the baby's potential to move caregivers. This establishes a safe space in which the infant then can begin to seek more direct mastery in the outside world.

CALL OF THE WILD

Almost all parents feel the urge to stick out a tongue in hopes their newborns will imitate them or to tickle their babies' bellies in search of a giggle. As I have written before (Marks-Tarlow, 2010), parents, by issuing the call to play, can follow a universal instinct wired deeply within the nervous system of most mammalian species and even a few birds and insects. While arising independently more than once during evolution, the instinct to play went hand in hand with the attachment system and the care circuit, discussed in the last chapter. Not only was play a major form of bonding between parents and their offspring throughout the animal kingdom, but play also went hand in hand with the open wiring and experience-dependent maturation of the mammalian brain (Panksepp, 1998).

In most species, the urge to play occurs within a critical window during the juvenile period (Beatty et al., 1982). For example, with meercats (see Figure 4.3), the impulse toward play fighting begins just before weaning and peaks at 25 to 45 days of age and relates to normal social and sexual development.

Play in humans resembles play in other mammals in also having a critical window for normal development. As with many other mammalian species, rough-and-tumble play during the early childhood years appears to be especially related to cognitive capacities to settle down and focus attention. This led the neuroresearcher Jaak Panksepp (2008) to suggest that all early elementary school classes should begin each day on the play-

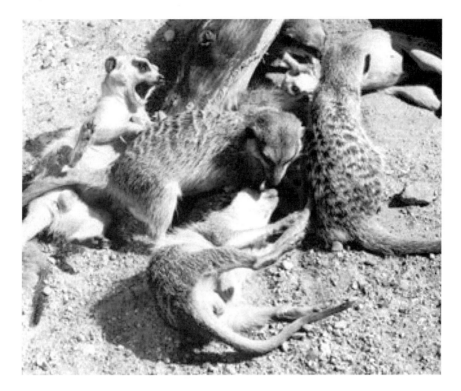

Figure 4.3. All social animals play like the meercats in this picture, and the play is mostly in the rough-and-tumble form of play fighting. It is easy to assume that this provides practice and skills for later fighting. But this is too simplistic. There is a host of hidden functions of play, especially related to emotional regulation. For example, with rats, early play fighting is preparation for later sexual relations.

ground. Panksepp sees running, romping, and grappling as a preventative measure against increasing diagnoses of attention-deficit disorder amid a backdrop of decreasing interest and funding for physical education.

When animals are meant to play but do not do so, whatever the reason, consequences can be severe (see Figure 4.4). They can wind up with severe behavioral, cognitive, emotional, and behavioral deficits. As described in the last chapter, Harry Harlow raised monkeys in isolation and deprived them of play. Many developed habits of severe rocking, thumb sucking, or other signs of self-soothing in response to separation anxiety. During adulthood they failed to develop normal social and sexual relationships.

According to Dorothy Einon (1980), isolated dogs that are deprived of play will actually walk into fires and demonstrate other severe learning

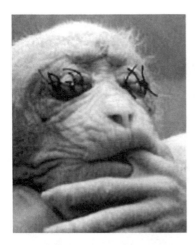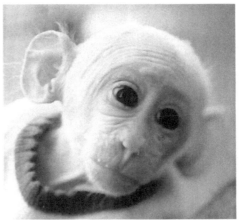

Figure 4.4. Britches, a baby stump-tailed macaque, was rescued by the American Liberation Front from a University of California, Riverside, laboratory in 1985. Clearly traumatized by having his eyes sewed closed for a research experiment, we see Britches self-soothing by sucking on his own fingers before treatment. After treatment, he is in a much more relaxed and open posture.

defects as adults. Einon's own experiments involved rats raised in isolation, without play. As juveniles, rats are creatures so fond of play that play becomes its own reward. This is demonstrated by their eagerness to learn a maze if permitted to play afterward. Rats deprived of play are behaviorally very active, if not frantic. Yet they cannot harness their activation effectively, such as removing an obstacle by pushing or pulling a ball out of a tunnel for a food reward. Rats deprived of play take a long time getting used to novel environments. They frequently struggle with memory tasks. Their behavioral style is inflexible, and they have difficulty stopping or reversing courses of action that do not serve them. Einon concluded, "I started by asking what the functions of play might be. I now believe play is not simply practice for later social interactions, but that it affects the versatility of adult behavior and the animal's ability to learn. The young rat becomes a more intelligent adult because it plays" (p. 936).

Stuart Brown (1998), a psychiatrist at Stanford, is a contemporary researcher who stumbled into a professional focus on play after unearthing a chilling example of its importance. As a psychiatric resident in 1969, Brown worked within prison settings, conducting clinical interviews on 26 young incarcerated murderers in hopes of finding common developmental threads. At first, Brown was puzzled by the highly diverse backgrounds of these felons. They came from such different social classes, ethnicities, levels of trauma and deprivation, as well as varying opportunities in life. Then Brown came across a single factor that these highly violent, antisocial men appeared to have in common: the absence of normal play during childhood.

THE PLAY OF IMAGINATION

We humans differ from other species that typically cease playing outside of their critical developmental window. People often continue playing right into adulthood. Sports like tennis or squash, hobbies like bridge or gambling, and virtual gaming adventures like World of Warcraft or Wii all compose the playground for adults. A strong connection between play and creativity leads many businesses to sport basketball hoops and other imaginative props. A connection between play, stress reduction, and physical resilience leads many holistically minded doctors to pre-scribe playful activities for adults (see Figure 4.5). Meanwhile, cross-word puzzles are the latest cure for preventing memory problems during old age (see Walker, 2005).

Along with its extension throughout the life span, human play differs from that of other species in another significant aspect. Beyond the rough-and-tumble variety common to other mammals, human play also diverges into symbolic realms and imaginative landscapes. Imaginative play is so im-portant developmentally for children that its absence during peak years, roughly between 3 and 6, is often diagnostic of a variety of problems (Brown, 2009), from specific developmental delays to severe autism.

Children's early creative play coincides with the development of sym-bolism through language. To a young child the world is a shiny, magical place, and language expands opportunities for the play of imagination, of-ten through imitation of adult roles (see Figure 4.6). Initially young chil-dren enact their conceptual understanding in physical form. When his mother's glasses case serves one minute as a microphone and the next as a cell phone, Tommy communicates his embodied knowledge of these objects. Whether or not these enactments initially are accompanied by a verbal stream, as Tommy grows, words will eventually enjoy a special place in his dramatic play.

According to Piaget, fantasy gets increasingly subjugated to constraints of reality as children shift from early sensory-motor play, through mastery play, to symbolic play, and finally to games with rules. Smilansky (1990) ex-panded Piaget's system into social realms: (1) functional or exploratory play, a sensorimotor foundation to learn about the physical and social world; (2) constructive play, a more active somatically based engagement with the world where children combine elements like blocks; (3) dramatic play, where reality is imbued with imagination and objects serve a metaphorical function (e.g., a stick becomes a sword); (4) sociodramatic play, a more complex form of dramatic play with implicit rules and multiple

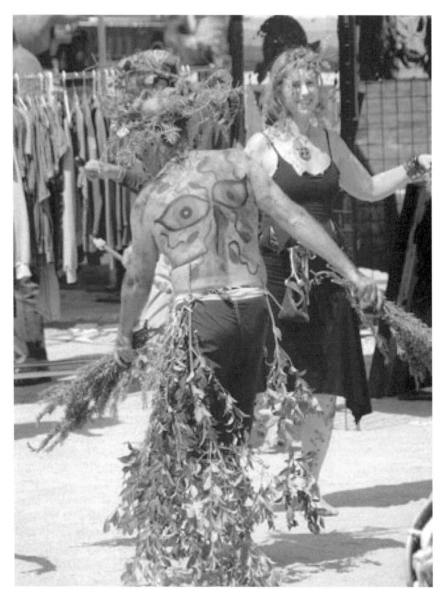

Figure 4.5. Just as the play of children is often serious business, sometimes the play of adults goes beyond entertainment or diversion. This man has costumed himself in accord with nature as part of a troupe of medicinal dancers as inspiration to others during an Earth Day celebration in Topanga, California, April 22, 2011. Here, adult play carries the important message to pay attention to the needs of the Earth. (Photo by Gene Blevins/LA Daily News)

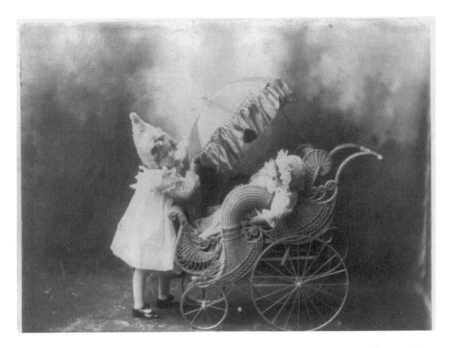

Figure 4.6. This photo, entitled "Baby Journeyings" was taken in 1900. By playing with dolls in baby carriages, this child imitated adult roles and activities. Throughout history and across the world, children love this form of play, and it is a major way they absorb cultural values and practices. (Photo copyrighted by S. Ford, Johnson & Co., Chicago)

players organized around a common play theme; and (5) games with rules, the most highly organized form of cooperative play, characterized by explicitly defined rules.

These categories reflect an increasing complexity as the left-brain competencies of language, logic, narrative, and conceptual self-awareness develop in the second year of life to combine with the right-brain foundation of affective processes and embodied self-awareness set in place by the early attachment system. As play becomes increasingly symbolic, social, and imaginative, it moves from implicit, preconscious, and nonverbal roots to include more explicit, conscious, and verbal elements. While still facilitated by safe attachment and primary-caretaker involvement, children's play develops in opposite directions simultaneously—toward greater autonomy as well as toward fuller coordination with others.

The seduction of our symbolizing side may easily give a false impression that play emerges from higher cortical capabilities. This is not the case, as demonstrated dramatically by Panksepp (1998) in a striking experiment. Panksepp's lab compared the play of normal rats to that of rats whose cerebral cortices were surgically removed. Undergraduate students were asked to observe and record the behaviors of the two groups, as well as to guess which group of rats was normal and which excoriated. Invariably the students guessed wrong, consistently mistaking the invigorated, boisterous antics of decorticated rats for normal ones, while the subdued behavior of rats whose brains were intact appeared less healthy.

Certainly humans love to use higher-thinking centers to continually innovate interesting, more sophisticated games. The cutting edge of technology often manifests in this way. The bright side to this is thrilling virtual play, while the shadow side includes nightmare visions like *The Matrix* or *Inception*, where play turns deadly or technology entraps rather than frees and expands our worlds. Yet like all other emotional and motivational circuits, the urge to play derives from primitive brain structures originating from the brainstem and subcortical areas. By contrast, the cortical level serves only to register, modify, or transform these deep urges, not to create them.

If the urge to play is so ancient and deeply wired into the brain, beginning well below any symbolic content, then what is its primary purpose? To address this issue in greater detail, the section to come has another animal tale to tell.

MONKEY SEE, MONKEY DO

Three juvenile patas monkeys are at play in the jungle. All three run up to a tree and begin climbing the trunk until they reach a long, horizontal branch. One after another, they inch out toward its end and then leap into space. Airborne for a brief moment, each lands on a large grassy patch of ground, quickly rises, rushes back to the tree, only to climb up and jump out into space once again. The group repeats the sequence at least 10 more times.

What is this monkey business all about? One obvious explanation involves the possibility that the monkeys are exercising the motor skills necessary to survive and thrive in the jungle as adults. We see this in the imaginary play of young human children who pretend to be doctors or astronauts, mommies or soldiers. Brian Sutton-Smith (1979, 1997) is particularly interested in imaginary social play that imitates adult perspectives and roles. Perhaps the monkeys practice climbing and leaping skills, which will prove useful in their future lives of seeking food, shelter and refuge from predators.

Yet Pellis and Pellis (2010) reported this episode of monkey play in order to illustrate a different function. These authors argued that if the juveniles were simply practicing motor skills they would maximize their safety by adopting a parachute stance in midair. To arch their torso and stretch their legs downward would ensure a soft landing. This is the position the Pellises claimed any "sane" monkey would assume. Yet these young patas adopted a different stance. At the height of the jump, each monkey raised its limbs laterally, assuming a spread-eagle position to land on its soft belly with what the authors call a "sickening thump."

Why did these monkeys act so crazily? Pellis and Pellis speculated that the belly flops taught the monkeys that having fun can involve pain, while conversely experiencing that pain sometimes feels like fun. Improvements in motor, cognitive, and social skills do arise indirectly through this kind of play. But its primary function appears to be emotional regulation—the generation of emotional responses plus expansion of the monkeys' tolerance threshold. By playing at the edges of regulatory boundaries in the zone just beyond the monkeys' safety and comfort, these animals become attuned to face uncomfortable events in the world. This builds their resilience to deal with uncertain circumstances, along with the flexibility to face novelty and risk with an attitude of adventure and gumption.

By giving monkeys the confidence to climb without falling, plus the experience of falling without dire consequences, play helped to dampen emotional responses to frightening, potentially painful situations (see Figure 4.7). Just as the limbic system is integral to the central nervous system, so is emotional calibration integral to behavioral, social, and cognitive development of all sorts. Translated into the ritual described with Sylvia, the positioning and repositioning of ourselves and the furniture in my office helped this young woman to tolerate her own "belly flops," while feeling motivated to get up again. In short, Sylvia and I were attempting to build a resilient base for life experiences through play, because, otherwise, the pain was intolerable.

PLAYING AT REGULATORY EDGES

Early play between a caregiver and baby also occurs at the edges of regulatory boundaries (Marks-Tarlow, 2010). Consider tickling, one of the earliest parent/infant games (as shown in Figure 4.8). This form of touch stimulates the baby, while enveloping her with her mother's presence. Sudden moves in and out of the baby's personal space, such as my lunging my head into the belly of Macy's baby (mentioned in the last chapter), allow parents to mimic the behavior of scary predators unexpectedly lunging in for attack. The high mutual arousal these games spark, including rapid oscillations between fear and excitement, stimulates the brain's reward circuits to provide a foundation for pleasurable flows throughout life.

Tickling takes place at that delicious edge where fear melts into pleasure. Babies are highly stimulated by early play, yet there is a risk of

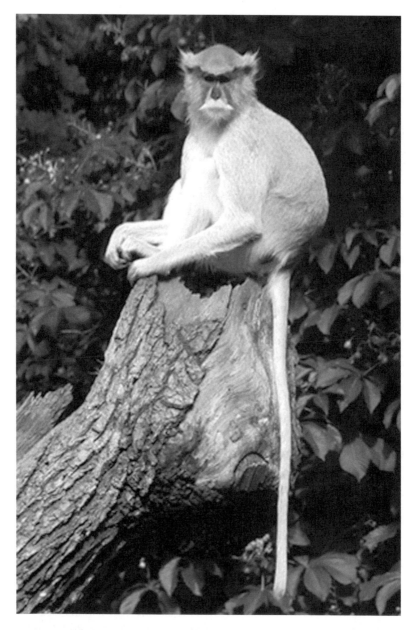

Figure 4.7. Patas monkeys are social, living in harem groups with up to 15 females and a single male who serves as the watchdog for the group. They prefer open grasslands, depending on speed for escape, but they can climb trees easily in which they tend to sleep, one monkey per tree, as protection against predators.

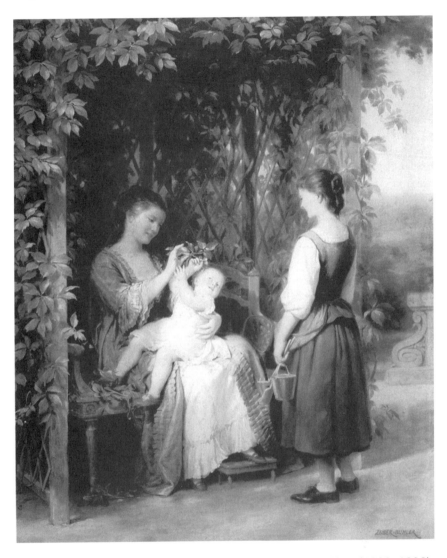

Figure 4.8. *"Tickling the Baby"* by Fritz Zuber-Buhler (1822–1896). Being nearly 200 years old, this painting implicitly communicates the universality and timelessness of the tickling phenomenon.

overstimulation if parents remain insensitive to their babies' tolerance thresholds for arousal. The line between pleasure and pain is a thin one. Play easily slips into abuse if the game is no longer mutual. The presence of a caring and responsive other is a key feature to this kind of play. If you have ever wondered why you cannot tickle yourself, the reason is because tickling requires the presence of another (Blakemore, Wolpert, & Frith, 2000). Like all early games, this one is played in intersubjective space.

To negotiate the delicate edge between pleasure and pain is a matter of timing. The timing of mutual coordination and turn taking is precisely where parental (not to mention clinical) intuition comes in. *Entrainment* is a term that physicists use to describe synchrony in timing called resonance (i.e., the tendency for two oscillating bodies to lock into phase and vibrate in harmony). Through entrainment, information produced in various areas of the brain becomes coordinated, even in the absence of spatially connected pathways (Buzsáki, 2006). In this way, the dimension of time becomes a primary means to forge new neuronal interconnectivity.

Play entrains people's bodies, along with their brain waves (Marks-Tarlow, 2010; VanderVen, 1998). We easily understand how a mother's and a baby's physiological processes become naturally coupled in the womb. Their hearts, brains, digestive systems, and even interior worlds are inseparably linked. Yet after birth, a baby still relies on its mother for emotional regulation and even regulation of physiological processes, such as sleep-wake cycles and digestion. Through attuned responding (Beebe & Sloate, 1982; Schore, 1994), early play between mother and child enables the complex coordination of interpersonal rhythms based on safety, trust, escalating arousal, and full engagement in positive emotional states. Early dyadic play promotes mutual immersion in Stern's (1985) "vitality affects" of excitement, joy, interest, desire, and curiosity.

THE PROTOTYPICAL GAME

If there is one game that is universally played among parents and children to capture the beginnings of social coordination and discourse, it is probably peek-a-boo. A baby's delight in "now you see me, now you don't" sets the rhythm for object constancy. Through the acts of appearing, disappearing, and reappearing, the baby internalizes a temporal sequence of positive engagement and disengagement, setting the stage for turn taking and "being alone in the presence of others," as Winnicott so beautifully phrased it. The game of peek-a-boo morphs into a more advanced version of hide-and-seek as the baby matures and becomes mobile (see Figure 4.9).

If there is one game that is universally played among therapists and patients, in my opinion hide-and-seek is the prototypical game, because it captures the flow of contact through rhythms of engagement and disengagement. Patients hide for many reasons, all emotional. Patients implicitly hide out of fear, shame, or guilt, and then they hope, dread, or expect therapists to find them. Patients may hide consciously and deliberately, as when addicts lie or psychopaths conceal information. Patients often hide when severely contracted and constricted with guilt or shame. Consider

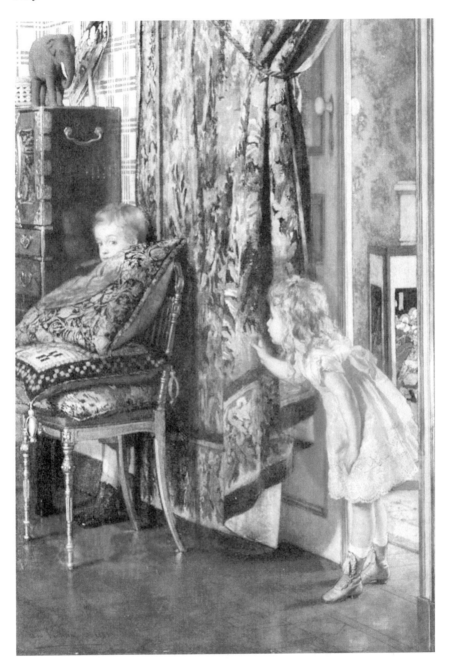

Figure 4.9. *"Hide and Seek"* by Jan Verhas.

the plight of Suzette, described in Chapter 2, who, after descending to the edges of the netherworld of prostitution, described herself as "living a lie." Suzette sought psychotherapy in order to address and break out of her life patterns. Yet she was so used to concealing the truth that Suzette may not have told me about her life circumstances had I not so quickly penetrated her veil of fear, shame, and denial. This was a case of conscious hiding, though more often patients seem to hide out of dissociated emotion. When this occurs, patients hide as much from themselves as they do from therapists and others who surround them. They then require our assistance to break through their own defensive barriers.

The impulse toward hide-and-seek is not limited to patients; it also comes from therapists, in what by nature is a reciprocal game. Every clinician must negotiate the dilemma of how much to reveal versus to conceal. There is no fixed answer to this question, but ever-shifting boundaries will depend sensitively on the dynamics of the moment. Do I speak of the horror I now feel in response to this patient's lapse of judgment? Do I simply let him read my emotion implicitly, as advertised with my facial expression and body language? Perhaps I go a step further in an attempt to actively conceal my emotions from the patient's detection, knowing how shame-prone that patient is as triggered by even the tiniest signs of disapproval? Recall the clinical tale of Bill in Chapter 2 who faked a suicide attempt in front of a young lady who was recovering from her own suicide attempt. If I could have hidden my disgust and contempt, I would have. For I became convinced that Bill left treatment prematurely precisely because he was able to read my emotions all over my face and body, and this was not helpful to him.

The role of self-disclosure during psychotherapy has been controversial from the start. Every school of psychotherapy agrees on the "seek" part of hide-and-seek. Virtually all therapists seek out their patients to help them feel known and as a means of knowing themselves more fully. That said, I recently learned of a marriage counselor who bases her technique on a 12-step model by telling couples, "I'm not interested in hearing your story. Every person either wants respect or adoration. You tell me which you want; I'll tell you what to do." But this is the exception; most of us do take great interest in what our patients have to say. Some of us are more active in the seeking pursuit. I, for one, often ask questions while making probing observations. Others assume a less vigorous stance by letting patients take more of the lead in coming to them. Most of us vary in how actively or passively we attempt to engage patients according to who the person is and what is happening in the moment.

By contrast to general agreement that patients should be sought out and fully engaged, the "hide" side of hide-and-seek is more controversial. Different schools disagree how much therapists should hide versus reveal of their full selves during psychotherapy. In fact, this may be one of the biggest differences between theoretical schools. Classical Freudian analysts conceal the self in order to grant plenty of room for patient projections. Gestalt therapists go to the opposite extreme by readily revealing the therapist's self in service of honest feedback and full contact. Self-psychologists track how the therapist's real self either facilitates or interferes with the emotional need satisfaction in patients. In cognitively oriented therapists, the therapist's self is often invisible and is considered a nonfactor in treatment. At the other extreme, relationally oriented therapists often highlight the importance of self-revelation, at least as it concerns authentic emotional exchanges with patients.

Despite the theories we hold, ultimately in the heat of the moment, it is clinical intuition that dictates when and how much we should reveal or conceal. While most clinicians believe it unwise to reveal many facts about their lives, at times a highly personal revelation that is delivered at an opportune moment can provide a turning point. Consider the case of Daphne, an accomplished doctor prone to depressive collapse into self-doubt and hopelessness. Daphne cultivated her career before she was ready or able to attend to her intimate relationships. As she crept toward her late thirties, Daphne began panicking at the thought that she would never marry or have children. At the same time Daphne's many years of personal psychotherapy allowed her greater openness while seeking a mate. As she began to date more, one day Daphne met Philip through a mutual friend. She was 39 at the time and he was 40. Neither had ever been married before. From the moment he laid eyes on Daphne, Philip was instantly crazy about her.

After going out on a couple of dates with Philip, Daphne announced during psychotherapy, "I really don't think this is going to work out. Philip acts *so* certain about our relationship. He is *so* positive about our potential together. But it's too soon. How does he know things can work out? Especially when I feel so uncertain? Philip doesn't know me yet. I'm not clear he even wants to. He's feeding me a line. His actions are based more on who he wants me to be than on who I am. I don't think I want to see him again."

"Can I tell you a personal story?"

"Sure."

"The first time my husband came to my door, he stepped inside my apartment and immediately declared his love for my taste in art. He stated that his taste was *exactly* the same. I was a bit taken aback by his strong feelings, but from that moment forward, he never wavered in his interest in me. That was nearly 20 years and two children ago. Many men experience full appreciation for a woman from the first glance. They are going by intuition. This doesn't mean they don't want to know us more deeply. What it sometimes means is that they are truly available for commitment and their hearts are sprung open from the start."

Daphne received my highly personal disclosure with great interest and a sideways cock of the head. She returned the following week to declare, "I had a huge insight during the week. *I have never been attracted to a man who was not depressed before*. I don't know what it feels like. I'm so used to being with self-absorbed men so wrapped up in their pain and the intricacies of their problems that they can hardly look up. My ability to understand these men and resonate with their suffering has always been my primary connection. Philip is so upbeat. He's so naturally outgoing. He's an entirely different guy from any I have ever been with. He's so outside my frame of reference. No wonder I automatically felt so much resistance and mistrust! As soon as I realized this, I started to relax. Now I'm in no hurry to leave."

Indeed, Daphne and Philip have just celebrated their third year of marriage along with the birth of a healthy, beautiful baby boy.

This game of hide-and-seek within psychotherapy is so primordial. I believe many become therapists out of a love for detective work and spy games, another more sophisticated variation of the hide-and-seek motif. Consider the early history of Jerome Singer, as revealed in *The House of Make-Believe* (Singer & Singer, 1990), a book that celebrates the importance of children's play for the developing imagination. Singer grew up in New York City during the early 1930s when boys liked to band together into "gangs" on the streets. Often while in one gang, Singer was "assigned" as a scout to spy on a rival one. Years later during World War II, Singer experienced later resonances of his early play when he received military training and once again was assigned to be a scout on assignment as a special agent in Military Intelligence. By subsequently becoming a psychoanalyst and researcher, Singer viewed himself as continuing his investigative work, albeit moving it from external to internal domains. And with this perspective, Singer identified with Sigmund Freud, whose own military experience became a rich source for metaphor. This is readily apparent within Freud's central concepts of intrapsychic conflict, defense, repression, alliances, and resistance (see Berkower, 1970).

As revealed in a recent paper (Marks-Tarlow, 2011), I became riveted by Singer's story due to the resonances it held with my own early history of play. I grew up in the suburbs of New Jersey where I, too, was captivated by the spy motif. Two television shows, *The Man from U.N.C.L.E.* and *I Spy*, inspired countless hours of imaginative play with my best friend. *Harriet the Spy* was my favorite book. And after reading Singer's account of his childhood, I suddenly detected these parallels between my own early history and the degree to which I remain a voyeur, "sneaking in" on patients as close as I can, now emotionally rather than physically. I remain drawn to "solving" the mystery of people's problems. This is highlighted within my specialty of helping to "free" people from the binds of creative blocks.

DEVELOPING EMOTIONAL RESILIENCE
THROUGH PLAY

Here is a clinical story of a serious form of play during psychotherapy that indirectly relates to hide-and-seek. Rita was the child of a depressive mother who took to her bed when Rita was about 3 years old. Rita's mother suffered a slow emotional and physical decline and then died just after Rita turned 6. Rita and her half-brother (they had the same mother but a different father), 10 years older than she, were subsequently raised by a well-intentioned but thoroughly absent father who struggled to make ends meet and was rarely around. The two became latchkey kids, left to fend for themselves. Not long after their mother's death Rita's half-brother approached his little sister in a bid for sex. Taking advantage of the huge age difference and Rita's desperate loneliness, her half-brother readily manipulated his little sister into an ongoing physical relationship consisting mostly in oral sex, but also involving full penetration at points. These affairs lasted several years, with the sexual forays conducted in complete mutual secrecy.

When Rita first sought psychotherapy with me, she was so thoroughly dissociated from her body that for many years she had taken to describing herself in the third person, either as "she" or by her own name, having abandoned the use of the word "I" altogether. I came to learn of Rita's history of sexual abuse by her brother as follows. One day, when I opened the door to my waiting room, Rita was sitting on the floor of my waiting room among a series of tiny figurines sprawled around her. The figurines appeared to be engaged in battle. I asked Rita to bring the figures inside my office and to recreate the scene. Thus began a slow progression of figurine depictions that moved initially from symbolic to quite literal depiction of the abuse over the next 6 months (an example of sandtray work with such figurines is shown in Figure 4.10). Through the play of these characters, Rita felt enough safety through emotional distance initially to depict and later to describe events she had literally and figuratively felt gagged from expressing.

THE NATURE OF DEFENSE

According to the hierarchy developed by Irving Maslow in 1943, basic bodily and emotional needs for shelter, food, and comfort must be met before higher-order desires toward growth and self-fulfillment can be considered. Maslow offered these ideas from an existential point of view, but they are supported by underlying neurobiology. A frightened, hungry cat will not eat, and a fearful, hungry, or cold animal will not play (Panksepp, 1998). A stressed animal siphons off too much energy from survival needs, leaving it unable to bring its full emotional, cognitive, and behavioral capacities to bear.

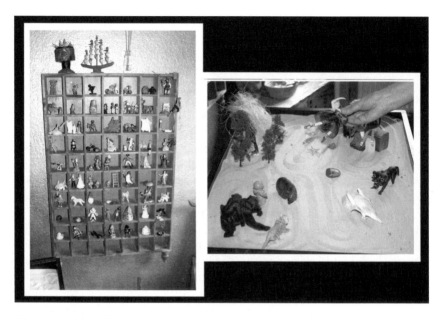

Figure 4.10. Originally developed as a mode of therapy by Jungian psychoanalysts, the sandtray is a dynamic, expressive way to play with symbols and metaphors within psychotherapy. Patients select pieces from among a wide range of miniatures in order to create scenes of relevance to their inner processes. Sometimes the journey takes on a mythological dimension; at other times it re-enacts an event from the past or it may bring here-and-now experiences to the forefront. No matter how the sandtray is used, this intuitive mode of therapy taps into creative self-expression and bypasses conscious deliberation. Photos by Kristina Walter, public domain.

Interpersonal neurobiology (e.g., Badenoch, 2008; Cozolino, 2005; Schore, 1994; Siegel, 2010) helps to shift how therapists conceive of the nature of psychological defenses. The cornerstone of Freud's early psychoanalytic conception of defense was repression. During the Oedipal phase of psychosexual development, children between the ages of 3 and 5 were thought to erect a repression barrier against forbidden desires to murder the same-sex parent in order to copulate with the opposite-sex parent. These forbidden impulses formed within the territory of the id, the underground backdrop upon which higher-order defenses were erected by the superego and mediated by the ego. Contemporary thinkers now consider dissociation and not repression as the primary psychological defense (Schore, 2009b). This concept emerges from trauma studies combined with increased knowledge about the dynamics of arousal within the autonomic nervous system. Whereas repression defends against *knowing* something, dissociation defends against *feeling* something too overwhelming to bear.

Allan Schore conceptualizes differences between repression and dissociation in psychoneurobiological terms. Here is a way to think about this. Whereas repression represents a *vertical split* between the verbal, conscious workings of the left hemisphere and the emotional, embodied, and experiential foundation of the right hemisphere, dissociation represents a more serious *horizontal split* between subcortical regions of the reptilian brain and higher-level limbic and cortical areas of the mammalian and neomammalian brain. Recall from the last chapter that rage and fear are aspects of the reptilian layer that evolved in the service of basic survival needs. This means that these primitive emotional circuits serve inherently defensive purposes against predators and environmental threats. When fear or rage circuits are habitually triggered, as when infants suffer repeated relational trauma or adults suffer from chronic work stress or physical danger during war, a horizontal split can occur that blocks access to higher-order social emotions or defenses, like rationalization and intellectualization.

This formulation aligns with Porges's phylogenic view of the autonomic nervous system, outlined in his polyvagal theory (Porges, 2011). He identified three levels of *neuroception* (i.e., implicit perception through the nervous system of the external environment): safety, slight danger, and severe danger. Each corresponds to aspects of our physiology that were developed during the evolution of the triune brain. Within the green zone of safety, we utilize an aspect of the mammalian circuitry related to social engagement, including relaxation and play. This circuit connects the heart, lungs, and brain stem to the striated muscles of the face and head, especially surrounding the mouth, giving rise to vocal gestures and speech. Porges's yellow zone of danger stimulates the sympathetic nervous system, causing us to become more vigilant of our environment in preparation for fight, active avoidance, or flight, allowing us to disengage socially. Finally, the red zone of extreme danger engages an aspect of the evolutionarily oldest circuit of the reptilian circuit. This circuit connects the brain stem to the lower centers of the gut, allowing us to respond to life-threatening circumstances through primitive means by feigning death and shutting down operations. Dissociation is a form of passive avoidance we engage in when all active paths become blocked, and the only "escape when there is no escape" becomes an inward one from experience itself.

Porges's hierarchy of arousal and response sheds light on how the care and play circuits go hand in hand for mammals. Whereas both realms of danger and life-threatening situations elicit defensive strategies, the realm of safety elicits spontaneous social engagement through eye contact, facial expression, prosody, posture, and other means of seeking connection to others, partly through the realm of play. Through nurturing instincts, parents protect their young from danger and simultaneously provide a safe zone in which play becomes a vehicle for social growth and self-development. Consider Porges's words here:

> Our physiology is a bi-directional system from our periphery to the brain, but our brain can also influence how our periphery works. Most therapies work on trying to get cognitions to organize the physiological state. And sometimes that's very, very difficult. It's often better or easier to try to get physiology to allow accessibility to cognitive structure. With that, I want you to think about play or group play as something extremely important in shifting physiological state. (2008)

Panksepp, who has done the lion's share of research on comparative animal play, agrees that new therapeutic approaches capitalizing on the positive emotions and proactive motivations of play could substantially improve therapeutic outcome, plus offer long-term protection against depression and related conditions (Panksepp & Watts, 2011). The incident with Rita demarcated the shift from the realm of danger to that of greater safety. Whereas the neuroception of danger leads to self-protection and defensive constriction, the neuroception of safety leads to self-expression and expansion. Rita began therapy from a purely defensive stance of fearful hiding and dissociative shutdown. From this platform of defense Rita's instinct to hide was initially not an invitation to be found, so much as it was an attempt to ward off demise by hungry predators in a "game" centering around power, control, and dominance. Over time, as Rita sensed the safety afforded by our relationship, she moved into the realm of self-expression through play. Her figurines allowed Rita to play a game that was no game at all.

THE PLAY OF POSITIVE EMOTION

Children's play is punctuated by exuberance of interest, discovery of novelty, passion to learn, intrinsic motivation to engage others, plus the sheer joy of being in the moment. Through play, the pain, risks, ambiguity, and uncertainty inherent in existence are all more easily and flexibly folded into experience without severe internal disruption. We saw in the patas monkeys how play became a powerful integrator of inner resilience with outer experience. Play maximizes the interconnectivity of the organism with context, the self with other, the past with future through an eternal present, the inner with outer processes, the receptive with active facets of physiology, and the expansive with reflective capacities.

Play is self-organizing, involving bottom-up immersion in the moment that is full of vitality. Play enables practicing and internalizing new rules, roles, and relationships. Social play teaches shared imagination, mutuality, agency, creativity, turn taking, give and take, social hierarchies, and leadership. As applied to psychotherapy, a play model widens the window of affect tolerance partly through affording a positive spectrum of emotions, motives, and experiences to integrate with the negative.

When people's positive sentiments outnumber negative feelings by three to one, they reach a tipping point beyond which they become more resilient in life and love (Fredrickson, 1998, 2001). Frederickson argued that while negative emotions narrow people's perspectives and keep them focused on a specific problem at hand, positive emotions broaden people's available repertoire of thoughts and actions as well as their behaviors. In this way, positive emotions grant more behavioral flexibility, allowing us to build intellectual and psychological resources.

I believe a central function of clinical intuition is to strike a productive balance between negative and positive moments in therapy. With issues of emotional regulation at the heart of psychotherapy (Schore, 1994), when patients feel overwhelmed, unsafe with their own experience, or cut off from negative emotions, therapists are careful to allow the full expression of negative emotions during sessions. But if the expression of distress becomes repetitive and lifeless, needlessly traumatizing, or heads therapy down the road of an impasse, intuitively therapists may be inclined to guide patients toward novel, more positive experiences.

This is what might be called the ordinary magic of therapy, where psychotherapy sometimes involves an emotional "sleight of hand" to move a patient's attention away from the obvious in order to produce something novel. Sometimes this shift in attention is top-down and intentional. Sometimes it is bottom-up, which is called sensory capture, when something in the environment is so compelling, we cannot help but notice it. Trevarthan (2001) wrote about the importance of joint attention as a precursor to intersubjectivity during development, when babies follow caregivers' eyes toward salient objects in the environment as a primary way to learn.

Therapists are masters of working with joint attention, especially at a metaphorical level. We pull our patients into seeing what we are seeing. They see us looking at them and then borrow our eyes to look at themselves. This is not the same thing as manipulating attention purposefully, because most of the time these processes work implicitly and automatically, as guided by clinical intuition, flowing holistically and organically from the shared intersubjective space.

Whether or not we are aware of it, through the "play" of joint attention, we help patients try on new inner perspectives the way they might go into a store and "try on" a new outer pair of clothes. Through play we bypass ordinary defenses connected with survival-level processes (e.g., fear and self-protection or anger and pushing away). Play occurs in a safe zone that inspires us to come out of hiding and come forward to engage with others and the environment. For patients to see an old topic from a new vantage point by borrowing our eyes carries the potential to bring them greater depth, much like using stereoscopic vision.

WRAP-UP

The play of psychotherapy is a vital part of how clinical intuition manifests at a moment-to-moment level. How and why psychotherapists play with patients will set the tone for sessions and determine the *feel* of the intersubjective process. Play is a vital instinct that is hard-wired into the mammalian brain. In this chapter, we looked at the interpersonal neurobiology of attachment to understand how the self grows, unfolds, and builds new structure through play. Freedom to play without inhibition or constriction is a key ingredient for joy, interest, passion, and vitality later in life. Just as children reveal their growing edge during play, so, too, do therapists. Because play is developmentally crucial to achieving cognitive, emotional, behavioral, and social flexibility and complexity, it remains a central part of the repertoire of clinical intuition.

Sometimes we therapists succumb to the instinct to play in order to lighten up the atmosphere. At other times the intuitive urge to play models an open, nondefensive attitude toward ourselves and others. Whether initiated by the therapist or patient, the instinct to play encourages the experience of fun during experimentation with new possibilities. The invitation to play is a bid for connection that allows coordination and turn taking. The capacity to play always signals safety in the room, and safety is necessary for novel expression and new coping to emerge.

Through play, we use our clinical intuition to feel our way into the unique contours of each person. Through the play of language, we find special terms reserved for each patient alone. Through the play of different expressions across our face, the idiosyncrasies of special greetings and innovation of unique rituals, we cocreate meaning that is carried only within this particular relationship. At implicit levels, we play with our focus to gently guide the focus of our patients toward new directions. At explicit levels, we play with how we frame and assign meaning to our patients' narratives, all in service of new hope, healing, and growth.

To bring home the themes of this chapter to your own clinical practice, consider the following:

- How does the game of hide-and-seek relate to your own brand of psychotherapy? Which patients hide? How do you seek? How do you hide?
- What is your stance on self-disclosure broadly? Do you think that therapists should reveal the content of their psyches and lives to patients? Do you hold a general position on this matter or do you ascribe to more of a case-by-case determination? If your self-disclosure is case-specific, how do you discern when to disclose and when not to?

- If you believe it is okay to be "found" by patients, what do you reveal? Inner states specific to relationship dynamics? What about your own attachment or developmental history that gives rise to these states and dynamics? Have you ever revealed circumstances or events from your own life? If so, how has this worked out?
- Aside from your own variations of hide-and-seek, what other games or ways do you and your patients play during psychotherapy?
- Here is one game I especially like to play. I take what I call "therapeutic license," akin to the poetic license taken by writers. I wave my magic therapeutic wand in order to change some facet of reality. This is not unlike a thought experiment in science, such as Einstein's proclivity to ride a light beam or drop with gravity in an elevator. By suspending certain existential truths, it can become easier to cut beneath the surface. For example, let's say a patient is considering leaving psychotherapy due to a scarcity of funds. I might take therapeutic license to magically eliminate money from the equation. By then inquiring whether the patient still wants to leave treatment, I can find out what lurks beneath circumstances, logistics, and excuses.
- Are there some ways you might take therapeutic license? More broadly, how might you play more freely within your practice to explore new frontiers?

Perhaps the reader has detected my love of humor by this point in the book. The next chapter examines the role of humor more directly in psychotherapy.

CHAPTER 5

Survival of the Wittiest

*A person without a sense of humor is like a wagon without springs.
It's jolted by every pebble on the road.*
—Henry Ward Beecher

*Imagination was given to man to compensate for what he is not; a
sense of humor to console him for what he is.*
—Francis Bacon

ALONG WITH ART AND SCIENCE, humor was considered by the late psychologist Arthur Koestler (1964) to be the third pillar of creativity. To create a joke is to bring together disparate things in a novel way. To understand a joke is to connect with the sheer pleasure of solving a little problem. Frank Howard Clark once commented, "I think the next best thing to solving a problem is finding some humor in it." Implicitly humor brings a sense of play and openness into relationships that can be invaluable to their fabric. Within psychotherapy, through clinical intuition we navigate the rhythms of humor. Whether initiated by the patient or therapist, humor offers an invitation to play within intersubjective realms, while communicating implicitly about the nature of the therapeutic bond itself.

Every therapist, along with each person, has a unique sense of humor, which intuitively guides some portion of our interventions. To share humor within psychotherapy can help to forge trust and positive experiences within an attachment relationship. To utilize and receive humor requires the idiosyncratic use of language that capitalizes on the highest capacities of the right brain. How and when clinical intuition prompts therapists to use humor as a powerful tool is the subject of this chapter.

It is no wonder that humor comes naturally into our offices, because humor is an important part of childhood play right from the start of life.

As discussed in the last chapter, when a mommy tickles her baby's belly, she behaves like a mock predator pretending to violate the baby's personal boundaries, yet her real intention is to deliver fun and pleasure instead. Laughter, as it connects to this humorous act of imagination, is deeply wired into our brains subcortically. Laughter tunes into amygdalar regions, which are the arbiters of safety versus danger and deep processors of humor from the start (Watson, Matthews, & Allman, 2007).

In this chapter, I begin with a discussion of the evolutionary roots of laughter and humor to bolster the necessity of clinicians taking this topic seriously. I then shift to psychotherapy, where humor can buffer pain to within tolerable limits, provide safety to approach shameful topics, and help to diffuse aggression away from violent levels. Ample clinical examples are provided. Like any other tool, humor can be used for good or poor treatment, and in addition to covering its positive sides, this chapter also explores its misuses and even abuses. Within psychotherapy humor can be abused if dispensed in service of avoidance, numbing, dissociation, or humiliation.

WHAT'S SO FUNNY?

Franzini (2001, p. 171) described therapeutic humor as both an "intentional and spontaneous technique of leading to improvements in self-understanding and behavior of clients." This formulation acknowledges the important quality of *spontaneity* surrounding the production of humor. Yet this otherwise cognitive definition is limiting in two ways. First, the definition implies that humor is an intervention *produced by the therapist* in order to illuminate or otherwise change the patient. Yet as we shall see, humor is an intuitive form of play during psychotherapy that is often initiated by the patient. Second, Franzini's definition implies that humor has a *conscious impact* on patients, whether it is produced intentionally or spontaneously. I propose differently—that the use of humor during psychotherapy need not be consciously produced or even consciously recognized. Instead, humor within psychotherapy, including its close relative, laughter, involves primarily implicit, and not explicit, communication. Specifically, humor during sessions involves communication that surrounds and highlights the current state of the therapeutic relationship.

Whether initiated by the patient or by therapist, I suggest that humor arises intersubjectively from the relational unconscious. What is more, the primary function of humor is to signal, through enactment, an emotionally relevant aspect surrounding the nature or quality of the bond itself, whether indicating safety or danger, progress or impasse, crisis or breakthrough. For example, a patient evading topics and deflecting with jokes might indicate the perception of danger. By contrast, affectionate ribbing surrounding shared humor, even around painful issues, could indicate the desire for or safety of connection. Clinical cases sprinkled throughout this chapter provide other examples in detail.

LAUGHOMETERS

Robert Provine is a researcher who is interested in the social and biological functions of humor-related behavior. In the introduction to his book *Laughter* (Provine, 2000), he lamented that his colleagues all too often refuse to take this topic seriously. Yet ethological research reveals that laughter is built into the very foundation of the mammalian brain. Laughter is a closed circuit, like coughing or sneezing, which may be triggered by environmental factors, but whose form is specific to each individual and does not depend on experience (Panksepp, 1998). Laughter is shared by many social mammals, including some surprising ones (see Figure 5.1), a topic further explored later in the chapter.

If such a thing existed as a laughometer that could measure wit and mirth through the course of a day, I would guess that each one of us would display a unique pattern of humor and merriment. If we were to collect time-series data to measure the pauses between incidents of either producing or responding to humor, I further speculate that the fluctuations would reveal a pattern of consistent inconsistency across all time scales, whether measured in minutes, hours, days, or weeks. If so, this would be the classic power law, a nonlinear statistical distribution found throughout much of nature, including human nature (Marks-Tarlow, 2004, 2008a). Power laws signal *identity* by revealing what remains constant underneath and despite continual, often unpredictable, surface change. If our reliance on humor were to follow a power law, then as an aspect of personal identity, its fluctuations and unique exponent for each person would resemble power law exponents previously measured for self-rated self-esteem, along with feelings about our bodies (Delignières, Fortes, & Ninot, 2004).

Given the possibility that humor is an important aspect of personal identity, within clinical work I suspect that each therapist uses humor idiosyncratically as a clinical tool. Furthermore I surmise that each of us turns to wit or laughter more with certain patients than with others, and more during certain stages of treatment than during others. And if all of this is so, these rhythms of humor that punctuate each clinical hour are navigated intuitively, as we feel our way through the contours of intersubjective space and time.

TO LAUGH, PERCHANCE TO
COMMUNICATE

Whether patients have a sense of humor and how they use or abuse humor can be diagnostic. Humor involves the play of social imagination. And just as the absence of imaginative play can indicate autism in young children, so the inability to participate in the social reciprocity of humor can indicate autism or Asperger's syndrome in adults (Neihart, 2000).

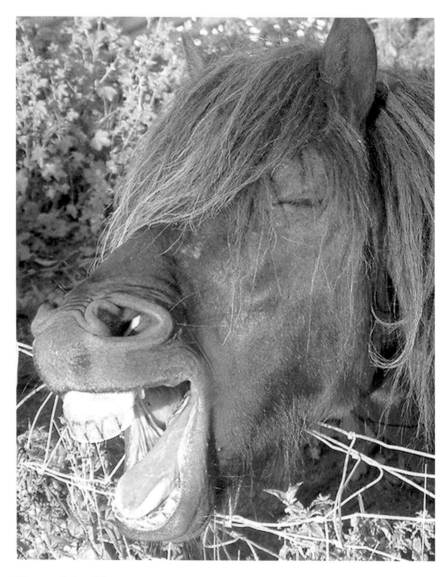

Figure 5.1. The photographer noted, "I hadn't met this pony before and as I put the camera up, this was his response!" Everything about this picture suggests an amused horse, but is the horse actually feeling this emotion or is this the projection of an amused viewer? (Public domain, courtesy of Rachel C)

Consider the words of Temple Grandin, a famed, high-functioning autistic woman who wrote eloquently in her autobiography, *Thinking in Pictures*, about what it is like to grow up outside of normal social patterns:

> When several people are together and having a good time, their speech and laughter follow a rhythm. They will laugh together and then talk quietly until the next laugh cycle. I have always had a hard time fitting in with this rhythm, and I usually interrupt conversations without realizing my mistake. The problem is that I can't follow the rhythm. (quoted in Provine, 2000, p. 35)

Allan Schore (personal communication) has suggested that symbolic humor is produced and appreciated by the high right-cortical hemisphere. The right hemisphere mediates spontaneous facial expressions in reaction to humor, including smiling and laughter (McGilchrist, 2009). It is the right hemisphere that understands the point of a joke (Coulson & Wu, 2005). Meanwhile, humorlessness in patients can indicate an overactive left hemisphere. This is confirmed by research showing that neurological damage to the right hemisphere often results in the literal interpretation of jokes (see Figure 5.2; McGilchrist, 2009; Tucker, Watson, & Heilman, 1984).

In my clinical experience, people who suffer moderate levels of anxiety sometimes appear humorless. Todd was a good example of a Type A personality who was efficient, productive, and had a strong work ethic. But Todd had a problem in knowing when to stop working. Even during social occasions or personal conversations, this young man, who seemed much older, tended to plod through endlessly. Todd carried tension continually in his face, including a jaw that perennially seemed locked down tight. Even without coffee, Todd was a "fine grind," by keeping his teeth grinding and his nose to the grindstone, indicating little time left to waste on silly jokes. Yet Todd's humorless style seemed more about sympathetic arousal and high pressure to race into the future than about anxiety per se.

I have noticed another type of anxious person who presents in the opposite way. Perhaps indicating a person more easily distracted by her own internal states, this sort of individual's very body seems to jitter naturally, as if caught in a perpetual laugh. Gilda, one of my former patients, was an example. As she got more nervous, instead of sweating bullets, she sweated out jokes, releasing tension while communicating implicitly, "If I can laugh at myself, and if I can convince you to join in, then there is at least one thing right and safe in the world. But only for a moment, until I crack the next joke." For people like Gilda who evidence an insecure, anxious attachment style, humor can become a central aspect of interactive emotional regulation.

Whether or not patients invite us to join in and whether or not we laugh along with them speaks volumes about the nature of the therapeutic

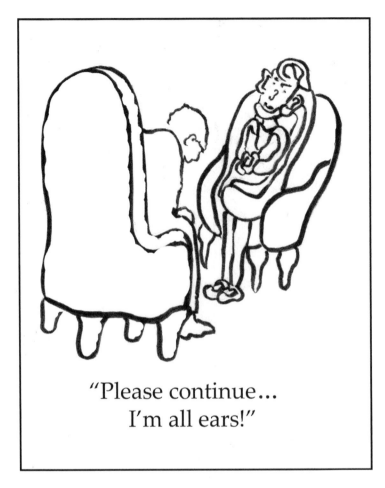

"Please continue...
I'm all ears!"

Figure 5.2. As the reader might guess from this cartoon, I can be quite literal when it comes to humor. In response to my husband's dry Bostonian wit, I initially struggled to understand when he was joking. In order to "get" his humor, I needed to be very conscientious about cultivating sensitivity to his social and facial cues. (Courtesy of the author)

relationship. Consider the social behavior of a patient named Blair, a young woman who laughed loudly every time I opened the door to the waiting room at the beginning of a session. Blair regularly continued her nervous laughing as she entered my office and passed alongside me to take a seat on the couch. During this extended period of time, I found nothing funny going on, and I did not find myself intuitively inclined to laugh along with Blair. In fact, I experienced the whole sequence as painful, which easily seeped into annoyance, which, to my horror, would crescendo into downright hostility on my part, all before Blair had even said a word.

To share a laugh during therapy can be an intimate moment. Yet with Blair, there was nothing shared or intimate about these laughing moments. In fact, had I laughed along, I imagine my participation would have been received as weird and completely "off." I imagine that implicitly I would communicate derision. By laughing when nothing was funny, I would be mocking my patient for her social awkwardness, making fun of her discomfort. Either that or I would be perceived as laughing at my own private joke that had nothing to do with Blair's presence.

True humor involves an intuitive understanding, if not mastery, of social rhythms. Because Blair's use of laughter did not involve humor at all, I regularly found that my access to my own intuitive side was completely blocked during these opening sequences. Instead, I was very consciously deliberating about how to respond. This included a lot of self-restraint to not express the anger and frustration, if not derision, I often felt. I could feel my lips drawn into a tight line, as if to ensure that nothing that resembled a laugh or snide remark would leak out. I received the solitary guffaws of my patient quite self-consciously, by bracing for the discomfort of the moment. My body perceived Blair's communication as a mixed message. Rather than as an invitation to share in the fun, I felt pushed away and even tricked, through being teased and left out of a gesture I would ordinarily feel motivated to join (who does not adore a good laugh?).

And all of this transpired in the brief few seconds at the start of psychotherapy. Meanwhile, intuitively I sensed this young woman was far too caught up in her own discomforts to be conscious of any implicit communications or emotionally laden reactions on my part. I also sensed Blair would never purposefully send or receive such messages. As a result, I regularly felt guilt at my own hostility, experiencing myself as assaulting my patient with feelings of discomfort and irritation. Along with these secondary feelings, Blair became the innocent victim in my eyes, and I the guilty perpetrator. Dooley (1941) wrote of the relationship between humor and masochism. Indeed Blair was quite self-effacing in style. And this gave way to yet another, tertiary set of feelings—hoping and attempting to empty myself of annoyance as quickly as possible, in order to "get on with" the "real stuff" of psychotherapy.

But I am sure the astute reader recognizes immediately that *all* of this *is* the real stuff. Much of Blair's work in psychotherapy surrounded the recognition of her need and efforts to reclaim her personal power in relationships. Insofar as the sequence at the beginning of each session mirrored the internal world of my patient, my own reactions partly revealed Blair's habit of regularly trying to empty herself of the bad feelings. This held especially true for despair and annoyance at her husband, whose avoidant style left him attempting to evade and vacate himself from true contact. Indeed, this was Blair's presenting complaint upon entering psychotherapy. She felt ignored, disrespected, and unhappy in her marriage, but she was unsure what to do about it.

When it comes to the realm of intuition, I am continually astonished by how much can be implicitly known and experienced without conscious thought. Consider the parallels between tiny moments in these opening minutes of our interpersonal ritual and Blair's larger-scale struggles with her husband and within herself. I am equally as astonished by how many words it takes to flesh out these micro-moments of implicit exchange! I suspect this ratio between the brevity of an implicit event and the length of its explicit description might be especially high whenever humor comes into the picture. Humor serves vital emotive, relational, and communicative purposes, partly by functioning as an intuitive bridge in the gap between lower, primitive subcortical circuitry and higher prefrontal areas, those pinnacles of symbolic sophistication.

In the case of Blair, laughter was an expression of defense, forming a barrier to contact rather than as an invitation into mutual engagement. There was little spontaneity about the laugh, which had become thoroughly scripted into our encounter. There was no humor behind the laughter, which instead signaled a kind of self-debasement. All in all, I experienced this opening ritual as quite stale, "inspiring" me to follow suit and lose my own spontaneity. Clearly, with so much transpiring during this first nonverbal (avoidance of) contact, such implicit exchanges are in themselves important topics of discussion. How and when such issues are brought to explicit light becomes itself a matter of intuitive feel.

LAUGH AND THE WORLD LAUGHS
WITH YOU

As a contrasting example to the use of laughter as a defense against contact, I would like to return briefly to the case of Sylvia from Chapter 4, the young lady who ritualized the start to every session by manipulating my furniture to suit her current state of mind. During psychotherapy with Sylvia, I laughed a lot, and I often experienced our mutual laughter as a way to bond in service of interactive regulation. As mentioned, Sylvia had informed me early in our treatment that her first therapist, whom she visited as a teenager, had little sense of humor. This was a deal breaker, because of the central importance humor took on to Sylvia as the gold standard of intelligence and wit.

Even in high school, Sylvia had been seriously attracted to comedy. She loved stand-up and aspired to be funny herself as a primary expression of her identity, as affirmation of her wit, and as testimony to her own high intelligence. From my point of view, that her previous therapist denigrated this side of Sylvia by interpreting instead of joining in the humor reflected either a personality mismatch between the two of them or poor clinical judgment on the part of the therapist (see Figure 5.3). Intuitively, I felt so clean about joining in and clear that my immediate love for Sylvia's wit, along with my willingness to partake in her wordplay and creative manipulation of ideas, was a major way that the two of us got into sync from the get-go.

That humor serves to align minds and brains is confirmed by the existence of laughter contagion. Although there is danger in laughter contagion if it serves to humiliate others during a mob mentality, there is a more innocent side to the phenomenon that partakes in delightful mutuality and even self-agency. As a little girl of 6 or 7, I regularly played a game with my best friend that illustrates this. One of us would signal the start of the game by declaring "Ha!" in a flat monotone. The other would respond with an equally flat "Ha!" Then together we would up the ante by declaring "Ha, ha!" which was usually enough to launch the two of us into a fit of uncontrolled laughter. These giggle-fests could last for minutes on end, including unpredictable outcomes like falling off the chair or winding up under the table. There was secret pleasure to be had if we succeeded in drawing a parent or another adult into the game, making them laugh so hard they would grab at their bellies or even rush to the bathroom to pee.

Provine (2000) documented some astounding epidemics of laughter contagion, including a famous episode in 1962 near Lake Victoria, in what is now Tanzania, at a missionary school for girls between the ages of 12 and 18 years old. The episode started when three girls began laughing so hard that they also cried while experiencing agitation. These laugh attacks lasted between minutes and a few hours at a time, with as many as four episodes in a day. The symptoms quickly spread to 95 out of 159 students. The crisis reached the point where the school was forced to close its doors for a period of months.

But things did not stop there. The afflicted girls sent home served as agents who spread the laughing epidemic still further. By the time the incidences abated approximately two and a half years later, a total of 14 schools had closed with more than 1,000 people affected in what was determined to have a psychogenic, hysterical origin. In the case of the laughing school girls, little appears constructive surrounding this sort of contagion. Later in this chapter Ramachandran's theory regarding the evolutionary origins of laughter helps to shed light on the positive side of emotional contagion.

SOFTENING INTO PAIN

Max Eastman declared humor to be "the instinct for taking pain playfully." In order to demonstrate this function of humor, especially as it relates to

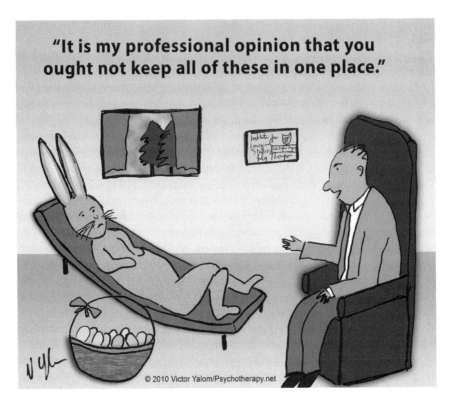

Figure 5.3. Just as there is no definitive rule for when and how to give advice to patients, there is also no definitive rule for when and how to use humor. Partly because they are such powerful interventions, strong cautions surround both enterprises. Timing is everything, and timing is always dictated by clinical intuition. (© 2011 Victor Yalom/Psychotherapy.net)

relational communication, I would like to relay the story of Sir James Matthew Barrie, the author of the famous children's classic *Peter Pan* (1904). Peter Pan is a lot more edgy, complex, and even tragic than the shiny Disney movie variety would have us believe. In *The Case of "Peter Pan," or the Impossibility of Children's Fiction* (1984), Jacqueline Rose especially made this case by observing Peter Pan's obsessive ruminations on "the question of origins, of sexuality, and of death." Indeed, there is true irony in the contrast between Neverland as a myth of childhood innocence and imagination versus Barrie's dark musings representing a retreat into fantasy in the face of early relational trauma.

Consider some facts of Barrie's early life. He was born the ninth of ten children in the Lowland village of Kirriemuir, in Forfarshire. Barrie's father was a handloom weaver, and his mother was the daughter of a stonemason. Trauma struck the family twice when two of Barrie's siblings died during infancy. Barrie's mother recovered by submerging herself in the rest of this large family. Barrie's mother loved to read adventure tales to her children in the evenings, including stories about pirates. But another tragedy struck, from which full recovery proved impossible. When Barrie was 7 years old, his older brother David died in a skating accident. David had been his mother's favorite child, and the accident proved the breaking point for Barrie's mother. She fell into a depression and took to her bed, never fully to rise out again.

Of all the remaining siblings, Barrie was the most distraught and affected by his mother's afflicted state of mind. Barrie spent endless hours trying to entertain, amuse, and rouse her from her depressive stupor. He became quite desperate in his attempts to gain her affection. He would, for example, dress up in his dead brother's nightshirt while imitating David's particular manner of whistling. In fact, Barrie became thoroughly obsessed with his mother, documenting these details in an adoring biography devoted entirely to her (Barrie, 1896/2011), which he published after her death.

Apparently Barrie's mother insisted that "good little boys don't grow up. They go to Heaven like David, where they can be with their mothers forever." In a horrific instance of mind/body confluence, Barrie never did grow up physically. His total height never exceeded 5'3". Although he sported a bit of facial hair, he never developed secondary sexual characteristics. Finally Barrie reputedly never consummated his own marriage, while also becoming thoroughly preoccupied with sadomasochistic sex, evidenced by kinky stories he wrote in his private journals. In response to so much early relational trauma, Robert Sapolsky (1998) speculated that Barrie suffered from psychogenic dwarfism, a hormonal growth disorder whose onset typically occurs between the ages of 2 and 15 in response to extreme stress—in particular, emotional deprivation.

Here we see both concretely, at a physical level, as well as socially and emotionally, how Barrie's life became severely stunted. Given this early history, it is little wonder that Barrie wrote about Peter Pan who lives in Neverland where boys never grow up, for Barrie never grew up himself. We easily detect resonances of early attachment issues and forms of play in the story of Peter Pan itself. Despite Barrie's deep emotional disturbance, or perhaps alongside it, he continually reverted to humor, both to represent trauma as well as to take refuge from it (see Figure 5.4). When it comes to the role of laughter in processes of both hurting and healing, the following line as drawn from *Peter Pan* is both poignant and haunting: "When the first baby laughed for the first time, the laugh broke into a thousand pieces and they all went skipping about, and that was the beginning of fairies."

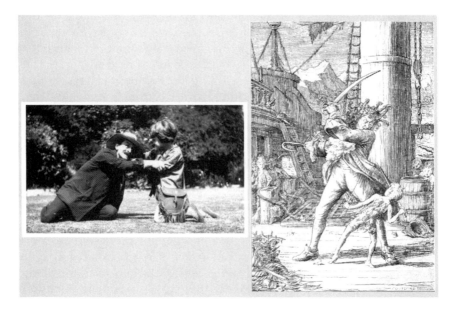

Figure 5.4. James Matthew Barrie playing Captain Hook and Michael Llewelyn Davies playing Peter Pan on the lawn at Rustington in August 1906, alongside page 188 portraying Captain Hook and Peter Pan in Barrie's book *Peter and Wendy*, published by Charles Scribner's Sons in 1912. (Photo credit unknown, presumably Sylvia Llewelyn Davies, art print by F. D. Bedford)

THE DARK SIDE OF HUMOR

In Barrie's case, we easily detect humor as an attachment-related communication both of desire and loss in response to Barrie's emotionally deadened, and lost mother. Barrie's humor served both as a refuge and a defense from relationally triggered pain. Within psychotherapy, humor is also used intuitively as a form of implicit communication regarding the state of the therapeutic bond. Humor-laden, implicit communications sometimes involve enactments designed to ward off expectations of being hurt, shamed, or misunderstood. In such cases, humor here, too, is used as a defense against true contact, including the experience of vulnerability this often brings. This certainly held true for Blair's solo laughter.

The potential dark side of humor, including sarcasm and mockery, easily gives humor a negative rap in therapy. While many have written about the positive uses of humor in psychoanalysis (e.g., Fabian, 1982; Mosak, 1987; Sands, 1984; Saper, 1988), Lawrence Kubie (1971) has warned of its destructive potential. Danger exists in using humor as a means to dilute contact, avoid pain, sidestep conflicted emotions, or collude with patient defenses. Children readily use laughter to humiliate and shame other children for differences or because of a lack of social graces. Unfortunately, the contagious nature of laughter often means that groups of children will join in the derision and chiding once someone starts, even if they are little inclined to start the incident themselves.

Provine (2000), one of the rare empirical researchers on the topic of laughter, concluded that it often serves as a social signal of dominance or subservience. After failing to produce many laughs under laboratory conditions, Provine and a bevy of undergraduate student assistants went into shopping malls and other public arenas to track and study the occurrence of laughter within normal social discourse. Under these naturalistic conditions, the group continually found themselves surrounded by laughter. Surprisingly, only 10 to 20% of pre-laugh comments were estimated by the research assistants to be even remotely humorous. Instead, laughter tends to serve as a form of social punctuation. Laughs follow gender patterns, with girls laughing more often than boys, and boys evoking more laughs than girls. Laughs tend to come at the end of statements, and the temporal segregation of laughter from speech provides evidence that different brain regions are involved in the expression of cognitively oriented speech versus the more primitive, emotion-laden vocalization of laughter.

Provine drew on ethnological studies to document the flexible, strategic use of laughter for displaying hierarchical structure within particular cultural contexts:

> In southern India, men belonging to a lower caste giggle when addressing those of a higher caste. Other aspects of "self-humbling" are well developed among Tamil villagers of low caste (Harijan), but are exercised only when dealing with powerful persons of higher caste. When dealing with a land-lord, for example, a Harijan may giggle, speak with unfinished sentences, mumble, appear generally dim-witted, and when walking, shuffle along. Yet this same Harijan may suddenly become shrewd and articulate when dealing with less powerful people. (p. 30)

The use of humor to establish dominance or to express submission reinforces its darker side and negative uses (see Figure 5.5). Indeed, a mocking, sarcastic tone rarely has a constructive role during psychotherapy. But even here, every rule has its exception, as I demonstrate next in the tale of a psychology intern, Elizabeth Lutz, who effectively used mock disdain intuitively to shift dynamics within a group of low-functioning, highly resistant patients. Lutz was serving as a counselor during a weekly group meeting at a residential program. Her job was to help the low-functioning members learn to live independently within a large apartment-complex setting. This was the first group meeting following the New Year, and there were only a few individuals present, as many members were still away on vacation. Those who were around had been in the program for at least 4 years, coming very regularly to the group, although Lutz had not seen some of them for months.

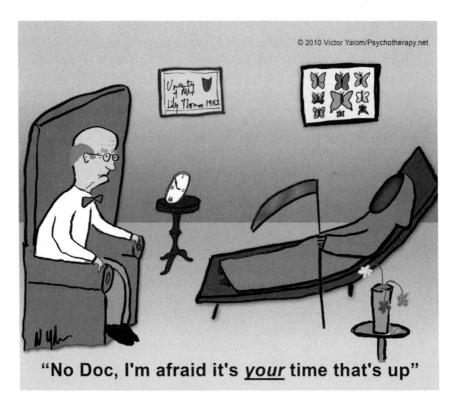

© 2010 Victor Yalom/Psychotherapy.net

"No Doc, I'm afraid it's _your_ time that's up"

Figure 5.5. Power differences between therapist and patient can be painful to patients, especially if power has been abused in the family history. To declare the beginning and end of a session is often a place where therapists reserve the full right to power. This cartoon reverses the picture by upping the ante and elevating the patient's power, in the case of the Grim Reaper. This elegant reversal is funny partly because it accords with the existential truth that we therapists are never really in control of much, plus a greater authority sometimes does sit in the chair opposite to us. Reversal is an important aspect of humor that is particularly relevant to psychotherapy because people often seek treatment to reverse conditions over which they feel helpless. (© 2011 Victor Yalom/Psychotherapy.net)

The residents met to speak about problems and receive input geared toward solutions from other group members. But this night was different. Lutz immediately sensed that all five participants were locked into defensive patterns, while resisting addressing their problems. In fact, even before Lutz arrived they appeared to be busily denying having problems at all. When the fledgling therapist sat down to join the group, Lutz announced a plan to talk about goals for the upcoming year, an idea that met with groans and eye rolls.

The most vocally resistant person was Natalie, and Lutz chose Natalie to begin the evening. This thirtysomething woman had been in the program for many years. Lutz felt instinctively drawn to addressing Natalie's patterns of resistance, which seemed to be blocking her further progress. In general, Lutz tended not to be directive in group, shying away from choosing the topic or who would speak. But during this particular evening, Lutz's intuition took her elsewhere. She continually surprised herself, first by singling out Natalie for group attention and then by picking out one of Natalie's goals—to be in the outreach program—and asking her point-blank how she had *not yet accomplished* this goal. Lutz was downright shocked at herself. This kind of negative phrasing was something she would ordinarily stay clear of. But on this evening Lutz's clinical intuition called out for a different technique.

Natalie answered Lutz's challenge by making comments so vague in content that nobody else in the group had any idea what she was talking about. Natalie had said, "I didn't tell people what I was doing, so I thought I was being independent. But it turns out I was wrong and wasn't supposed to do that. It would have been more independent for me to let other people help, like what I'd been told to do."

Lutz asked in a gentle but joking tone, "Does this have anything to do with an incident of flooding that I happened to hear about?"

Natalie looked surprised. "How do you know about that?"

"You should know by now that I know everything. . . . So why don't you explain what happened to the others? They might not be quite so well informed. In fact, they're looking pretty puzzled by what you just said. Take a look around at their faces."

Christine piped in: "Yeah, what are you talking about?"

Natalie appeared to look toward Lutz for permission to explain because the group has confidentiality rules. Lutz encouraged her with, "This is *your* story to tell. Tell it if you wish. *I* certainly think it's pretty funny!"

"I guess you're right. Looking back, it is funny!"

Natalie launched into the tale of moving from her last apartment in the complex into a new one. She had been told to let the manager, Helen, take care of the move. But Natalie confessed that she had been so excited about moving that she couldn't wait and so she got her friends to help instead. When mentioning this aspect of the story, initially Natalie was poised to defend her own actions, but then she sheepishly switched gears to state that her actions had been premature.

Realizing that Natalie was leaving out a critical bit of information, Lutz prompted, "Wasn't there a bit of water?"

Natalie laughed. "I'll say. The toilet flowed over!"

"And what did you do in response to that, Natalie?"

"I closed the door to the bedroom so it wouldn't get out into the hallway."

"I bet that worked about as well as it does in the movies," Lutz countered.

Natalie looked at Lutz sideways with a grin. "You got that right!"

The entire group burst into peals of laughter.

"So what happened next? How did you get help?" Lutz was aware of bringing Natalie back to task by confronting her defenses and habitual patterns of hiding the truth, which kept Natalie from clarity, both in her relationship to others and in her relationship to herself.

"I told the leasing office there was a leak . . ."

"Ahhhhhhh."

"I didn't know they couldn't do nothin' without Helen's permission."

"Hmmm. . . . Oh really? And how long have you lived here!?"

"Well, okay, the truth was that I really didn't want to tell Helen. I knew she was gonna get real mad."

"So you didn't tell the leasing office there was a flood?"

"No, I just told 'em there was a leak."

With mock sternness, Lutz implored, "So you didn't really tell *anyone* what was going on?"

"Nope, I didn't tell nobody nothin'."

"Then what happened?"

"They called Helen on Monday. You shoulda seen her face!" Natalie starts to laugh. "I never want to see that look again!"

Christine, the group member who had originally asked for clarification, laughed so hard she started falling out of her chair, murmuring along the way, "I just keep seeing the toilet flooding over!"

"No," responds Natalie, "it's Helen's face that's so funny!"

"No," rebuked Christine. "It's the toilet! I see the toilet!"

"I'm telling you—you never want to see Helen look like that again!"

"Have the carpets dried yet?" Lutz asked, shifting gears in hopes of solidifying the ground (so to speak).

Natalie started to laugh again. "Yeah, the carpets finally dried," she said.

"Ah . . . so, looking back, how would you explain what happened, Natalie?"

"I was too excited to do what I was told. When things went wrong, I made it all worse, because I didn't get the help I needed."

"And what did you learn from all of this? Is there something you would do differently to change your behavior in the future?"

Without missing a beat, Natalie responded, "I intend to be more honest."

Everyone seemed satisfied with this exchange, and so the group moved on to another person. The story above illustrates how Lutz used humor to break through Natalie's defensiveness around being honest and owning her mistakes, both with the group and with Helen, the apartment manager. Lutz continued to use dark humor in what followed.

Suddenly Natalie interrupted the next person who had started explaining her goals for the New Year, interjecting, "I'm gonna go to the pier tonight with my parents. We're gonna celebrate my big move together."

Responding to her enthusiasm rather than to the interruption, Lutz asked, "And are you going to play skee ball?"

"What's that?" Natalie asked innocently.

Lutz glanced at Natalie, and then gave her a disgusted sniff while raising her eyes and eyebrows with a smirk as if to say, "I won't even deign to give you a response or look at you." Meanwhile even Lutz was again shocked at her own behavior as a therapist, which seemed so totally out of character.

But Lutz proved to have her finger right on the pulse of the group. Natalie responded with an uproarious laugh. This caused the whole group to roar with delight in turn. Meanwhile no one wanted to tell Natalie what skee ball was. It was as if everybody was complicit with the positive side of Lutz's gesture—the invitation to enter the huge, exciting world outside in order to find out for herself. And even with her own question about skee ball remaining unanswered, Natalie nonetheless smiled, relaxed, and turned her attention fully to the next group member.

By rolling her eyes and thereby mirroring the members' gestures at the start of the session, Lutz used humor initially to join the group where it started, in order to break the tension that was evident in the initially resistant group. Later, Lutz playfully used a similar kind of mock humor to set a boundary around Natalie's interruption. Again her humor served to further bond the group. A key aspect of clinical intuition involves feeling your way through the intersubjective thicket to determine when humor serves to deepen versus when humor serves to block the therapeutic bond and capacity for inner work.

The psychoanalyst Philip Bromberg uses the phrase "safe surprises" for those key moments of meeting between a therapist and patient where something new emerges. A safe surprise is also one important way to view humor (see Figure 5.6). A common cognitive theory suggests that the origins of humor are in expectations that are violated. As therapists, in order to keep things fresh, slightly unsafe, and continually new, we intuitively play on the edge of patient expectations. Elizabeth Lutz used humor unexpectedly and without precedent to continually violate the expectations of group members. In this case, a series of safe surprises helped everyone to drop their defensive stances, become more cohesive, and attend to clinical business.

Therapists have historically had a love/hate relationship with humor, jokes, and laughter during therapy. Some have eschewed the use of humor by focusing on its defensive functions to ward off true contact. Others have focused on it as a powerful intervention. These polarized stances implicate the power of humor as an intervention, whether in service of helping or harming things. There are no rules that can be applied in all cases about when, how, and with whom to use humor. In fact, there is

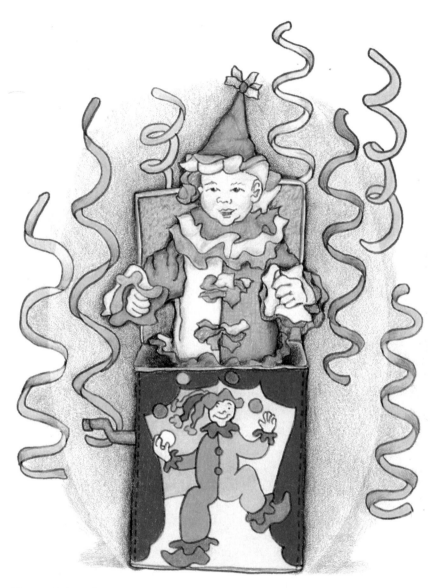

Figure 5.6. This drawing is an example of a safe surprise. Rather than to play with the Jack-in-the-Box, the child is part of the box. This reversal of what is outside versus what is inside not only makes for good humor, but also constitutes good psychotherapy. (Courtesy of the author)

something inherently violating about the very attempt to systematize, analyze, or prescribe the details of what naturalistically emerges unbidden and spontaneously as an act of interpersonal creativity.

Therapists should not stand apart from the process and get too analytical. Instead, they must immerse themselves in the process to feel their way through each moment. And all the while it behooves all therapists to heed E. B. White's warning, as expressed in the preface to *A Subtreasury of American Humor* (1941): "Humor can be dissected as a frog can, but the thing dies in the process and the innards are discouraging to any but the pure scientific mind."

HUMOR IN SERVICE OF
RUPTURE AND REPAIR

In Lutz's story, feigned mockery on the part of the therapist proved successful in breaking through patient defenses. In the case I am about to describe, my spontaneous impulse toward humor proved disastrous, revealing its potential to do harm. I wish to revisit a patient described earlier, Gus, introduced in Chapter 2 as the man who, at times, experienced himself as a woman. Earlier, this case illuminated the gap between explicit and implicit levels of therapy. You may recall that my gut reaction to Gus's request to help rid him of this experience was a complete protestation at a body level. Despite explicitly claiming he had little interest in self-exploration, Gus implicitly acted differently. Not only did he set up a first appointment with me, but also he wound up fearlessly pursuing in-depth psychotherapy for years.

As described in Chapter 2 and elsewhere (Marks-Tarlow, 2011), Gus's symptoms shifted and morphed along with our work together. The incident I am about to relate happened one day when Gus was describing the latest permutation of his experience as a woman. Frankly I forget Gus's specific comment that preceded my response (probably a case of traumatic forgetting on my part). What I do remember is that Gus asked me whether a very tiny detail of his condition seemed "weird." I am still horrified at my response, which I intended as a funny but comforting quip but which backfired so terribly.

I replied, "It's *all* weird!" I meant that the detail about which Gus was perseverating was no weirder than any other aspect of his broadly unusual experience. This was meant to be a reassurance that Gus had little need to hone in and pick at himself the way he was. But obviously this was not how Gus took my remark, which sounded to him instead like I was calling the whole of him *plain weird*. Needless to say, this mistake on my part was very hurtful. In the very next session, Gus declared that it was better for him not to discuss this sensitive side of his inner life any longer during psychotherapy. Fortunately we had built enough mutual trust that

Gus had the good sense and courage to let me know how he felt and to hang in there while we hammered out the pain and anguish.

My willingness to admit my mistake without hesitation or defensiveness, to talk about it openly, and to apologize for being so careless as to trigger such pain and shame proved a first in Gus's relationships. My ownership of responsibility for my part in our dynamic stood in sharp contrast with his previous relationships, especially his narcissistic mother or his current wife, who refused to talk about anything of emotional significance between them, much less take responsibility for her part in the dynamic. Despite Gus's vow at that point never to discuss his female side again, in the end, the episode proved a remarkable opportunity to go through rupture and repair. Ultimately the whole sequence solidified our mutual trust, allowing us to continue working at even deeper levels.

We both realized that Gus had worked through the episode thoroughly in light of a more recent occurrence. When Gus first came to see me, I asked if he had told his wife about his inner experience of feeling like a woman. Not only had he not told his wife, but at that point in time Gus could not imagine *ever* telling anyone about this aspect of his inner life. Gus believed he would lose his wife if he did so, and he held resolutely to this conviction for years. However, it all shifted, when in the wake of his heightened self-acceptance, Gus decided to reveal his innermost secret to a cousin. This occurred after his cousin had rebuked Gus for not sharing more of himself with her. She asked him point-blank about his "dark side," and Gus decided that it was time to disclose his deepest secret.

During our session, when Gus reported his most recent email exchange with his cousin, he said with a deadpan expression, "Laurie just wrote me an email declaring me the 'sanest' member of our family."

Upon hearing Gus's news, I burst into a peal of laughter. Almost immediately Gus joined in the hilarity, the two of us laughing together on and on. When we had finished literally wiping the tears off our faces, Gus said, "I asked Laurie's permission to tell you. I predicted to her that you would respond to this news with laughter."

"You were right! I couldn't help it. The irony is too beautiful, especially when thinking back to your longstanding fears that if you told anybody your secret, they would immediately reject you for being totally weird and crazy."

"Not only does my cousin think I'm sane, but she also mentioned admiring, if not envying, my form of adaptation. In fact, as she struggles with her own recurrent illness, and some really painful cancer treatments, Laurie admits wishing she could be more like me."

"You see, this is the beauty of having shared your deepest, darkest secret with another human being. Not only is she countering your worst fears, but despite your disbelief, she's giving you the highest compliment."

"It's all I can do to keep from dismissing my cousin's remarks immediately. What she writes seems so absurd!"

"Well, I'm here to tell you that they aren't absurd at all! I can see how you would appear ever so sane from her perspective. Precisely because you dissociate away from uncomfortable emotion, to her you appear level-headed, if not saintly. You remain understanding and compassionate to others and never seem to lose your cool, regardless of how much others lose theirs. All your distress gets tucked away so nicely, deep down inside, where it doesn't appear to hurt anyone, yourself included—very sane indeed!"

"Hmmm. I've been so caught up in feeling weird and freaky, this perspective turns it all upside down."

"Life often appears stranger than fiction. Sometimes all we can do is toss up our hands, surrender to the absurdity of it all, and keep on laughing."

In Gus's tale, our ability to laugh together about our previous rupture felt truly healing. In fact, the rupture itself now seemed terribly funny when juxtaposed with the story involving his cousin. Right from the beginning, Gus had taken a big emotional risk in telling me about his experience of feeling like a woman. He feared my responding to him the way the previous therapist did—by showing him the door and referring him out to a gender disorder clinic. This felt to Gus like "forget it; go somewhere else—you're too weird for me." Instead, I welcomed Gus into my office. Still, I was only a stranger. Had I rejected him, it would have hurt, but it would have been nothing like the risk he felt when he shared his inner life with his cousin. If Laurie had responded with revulsion and expulsion, Gus would have experienced this as intolerable. But beyond her acceptance, to have his cousin express quite the opposite—to be enthralled with Gus's coping, to consider it clever and a thing worthy of envy—was something he had dared not consider might happen.

Gus knew I would find this story unbelievably funny. That he was able to laugh long and hard with me was not just a quirk or a brushing off of serious business or another defensive reaction. To me, the capacity to laugh together in the wake of trauma indicates something else more fundamental, as I hope to reveal in the next clinical vignette.

LAUGHING OUR WAY TO SAFETY

When Goldie first came to see me, she looked frail, with her face pale and drawn, her body thin and tight. In fact, it appeared as if Goldie had stopped breathing altogether. Goldie's father had died suddenly and unexpectedly when Goldie was a mere 10 years old. Goldie had absolutely adored her father, who remained so high on a pedestal in Goldie's mind that no real man could compare. Only upon entering her late thirties did Goldie date seriously at all. And then she met Jake, whom Goldie perceived to be the man of her dreams. He was funny, smart and wooed her ceaselessly. After a romantic courtship of 15 months, the two tied the knot.

Two weeks later the fighting started and had not stopped since. In the subsequent years a side of Jake came out that took Goldie by complete surprise. She had not the slightest hint that Jake had the capacity to be so sarcastic, biting, aggressive, controlling, and unrelenting.

"I began wondering 'Who is this guy?'" Goldie explained to me, after many years of trying to chalk the problems up to various circumstances.

But the fighting continued and after a month, Goldie insisted that they go to couple's therapy. During that first session when the marriage counselor said to Jake, "Whoa, why are you talking to your wife with such a harsh tone?" Goldie knew she was in serious trouble. She wondered if she had made a mistake. But she hung in there, had two children, struggled with raising them, and then struggled with her health, getting a rare type of digestive disease, which was all-consuming and which had brought out the best in her husband, who himself had struggled with physical pain and health concerns his whole life.

Now years later, Goldie sought individual psychotherapy, feeling tired, confused, and depleted. On the outside, by all appearances, she had everything. But on the inside Goldie had completely lost her way by the time she found a path to me. I could see that Goldie was in a state of hyperarousal continually. It was hard for her to relax, even in her own home, because she never knew when the next criticism or attack would come. And on top of it all, her husband simply did not understand her concerns. He was an ex-heroin addict devoted to the 12 steps but very wary of emotion. He simply saw himself as "the way I am." To Jake, Goldie appeared "ungrateful" and "selfish" for not appreciating all his hard work and all that he provided materially.

Everything felt "like work" to Goldie, including her children, both of whom suffered from developmental delays. Goldie feared the worst. The more she worried, the more stressful became the home environment. Finally, the point came when both children were launched to school. The stage was set for Goldie to focus on herself. But on the very first day her second child was in school, Goldie fell into a state of unexplained dizziness, and it eventually got so severe that she became completely preoccupied with visiting specialist after specialist.

Given that none of the doctors found a physiological basis for her symptoms, from my end I took "therapeutic license" to declare this a "healing crisis." I spoke to Goldie about feeling metaphorically dizzy at not being so weighed down by the special needs of one or both children at home. I waited patiently. Slowly the symptoms diminished. During the first session that Goldie did not begin with an updated description of symptoms, here is what transpired.

"My husband and I had a really intense talk this weekend. He said, 'Goldie we're going to have to have sex at some point,' and this opened up a talk about intimacy. About how hard it is; how much work it feels like; how different it feels for each of us. I tried to explain my own experience. How lonely it is for me. How hard it is that Jake doesn't seem to understand my feelings. And, sure enough, all he could do was to go back into his song and dance about how hard he works to provide for us and how ungrateful I am."

"At least this was a conversation and not a heated argument."

"Yeah, that was different."

"You know, especially with your younger daughter diagnosed 'on the spectrum,' I've been thinking that your husband might have a similar condition. He seems so utterly incapable of getting inside of your head to feel the world from your point of view."

"That's so true!"

"You know, there are two kinds of empathy. One kind is emotional—Jake's ability to feel what you feel. The other is cognitive—Jake's ability to reason about your experience. That part he has. He knows you're unhappy, but because he's missing the feeling part, he makes up stories about why you're unhappy from his own point of view."

"Oh my God, you're so right! I'm having a lightbulb moment."

"You've not considered that his lack of empathy is actually a disability on his part before, have you?"

"No, I haven't."

"So then the question becomes, can you live with this?"

After expressing much sadness about the tragedy of this through a veil of tears, and then exploring together whether Goldie might get deep understanding from other sources, my intuition prompted me to say, "You know Goldie, no matter what, no matter who you marry, *there's always something really, really wrong.*" And Goldie looked at me with wide open eyes as if hearing this idea for the first time. Sheepishly she asked, "Is that really true?"

"Yes, it's really, really true. For everyone."

Then after a beat when we just looked each other straight in the eyes, suddenly and spontaneously, the two of us burst out into the deepest of laughs simultaneously. In fact, we both laughed so hard that again we were crying. And during the first semblance of a pause in the laughter, I took it upon myself to add, "And whatever that thing is that is wrong, it always feels like it could kill you." This, of course, only added to the hilarity.

Goldie summed up the importance of what happened by concluding, "You know, that's the first time in 8 years I've been able to laugh about my marriage."

And with this laughter came a breath of fresh air where none was to be had previously. Clinical intuition guided me to state what could have easily been experienced as highly controversial, if not stupid—first, that every relationship retains a tragic flaw; second, that we easily experience such flaws as fatal. In relationships as in life broadly, timing is everything. Only clinical intuition can guide us through these delicate affairs. Clinical intuition allows us to take social risks when we implicitly sense the moment is ripe. After Goldie released her externalizing defenses enough to relax into her own role within the marriage dynamic, intuitively I sensed the safety to inject a little grim humor to further loosen her idealism about how her husband *should act* and what marriage *should feel like*. My dark humor prompted Goldie to focus inside herself, on emotional challenges of how to make peace with her husband's flaws or alternatively to decide that she cannot. Perhaps the capacity to laugh about our relationship struggles is diagnostic of the capacity to retain perspective.

LAUGHTER AS A BOTTOM-UP RESPONSE

An increasing number of therapists are approaching psychotherapy from the bottom up or by working directly with the body and its response. Techniques such as somatic experiencing (Levine, 1997, 2008) and sensorimotor psychotherapy (Ogden et al., 2006) operate under the theory that trauma gets frozen and held in the body in the form of unexpressed emotions and incomplete actions. If this is the case, then no amount of top-down, talk therapy will touch this deepest level in which trauma is held. Patients are encouraged to reprocess their experiences by completing actions and discharging emotions that have been pent up. When a patient automatically jokes or laughs at the end of a sequence involving intense autonomic nervous system dysregulation, it can be a "sign" that the discharge of blocked or dissociated emotion is complete, that re-regulation has been integrated into the nervous system, and that the healing of that "piece" is complete (Ogden et al., 2006). And so it was with Goldie. After years and years of feeling victimized because her husband had no emotional empathy for her, the tables were turned. Goldie realized that in some critical ways it had been she who lacked empathy for him.

THE ORIGINS OF LAUGHTER

As mentioned earlier, Jaak Panksepp is a neurobiologist who for decades has been interested in the affective experience of animals. A number of years ago, along with a star graduate student, Panksepp made a remarkable discovery relevant to this chapter. If you take a rat into the palms of your hands, turn it over onto its back, and then tickle its belly, the rat responds by laughing. The laugh takes the form of a high-pitched chirp, at around 50 hertz, far too high for the normal human ear to detect. Perhaps this is why no one suspected that rats could laugh before, or maybe Panksepp was right during an interview he gave to the *American Journal of Play* (2010). Panksepp speculated that the field of animal emotions largely has been disregarded and underfunded because people do not want to believe that their emotional experiences overlap so thoroughly with that of animals (see Figure 5.7). Somehow this compromises human dignity. But like it or not, the realm of laughter is one we share not just with the "higher" primates but also with mammals as "lowly" as a rat.

Vilayanur Ramachandran (2011) hypothesized on why laughter might have evolved in the animal kingdom by setting forth what he called the False Alarm Theory. Here is an animal illustration. Imagine a leopard enters the territory of a troop of monkeys. Just as with humans, the right amygdala of the monkey is sensitively geared toward picking up danger. When on the alert, an animal will automatically cock its head to the left because danger is most easily detected in the left visual field. The first monkey to pick up the sight or scent of the leopard will instantly vocalize its fear with a scream. Because fear is contagious throughout the animal

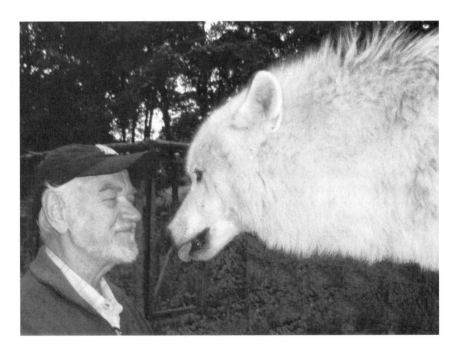

Figure 5.7. In this photo, Jaak Panksepp is kissed by a timber wolf. Rats and monkeys are not the only mammals to exhibit laughter. A form of "doggie laughter" has been described by the recently deceased animal behaviorist Pat Simonet. The laughter consists of a special kind of eager panting sound that can be discriminated from panting out of tiredness. Humans can simulate this play pant easily, and along with a properly conducted play bow, many dogs will reciprocate unmistakably with an eagerness to play. (Courtesy of Günther Bernatzky)

kingdom, the monkey's warning will be picked up and reverberate throughout the troop until all animals are properly alerted.

But what happens if a monkey makes a mistake about the presence of a leopard? Or what if the predator moves beyond the bounds of danger? There also needs to be a signal to the rest of the troop that the coast is clear. Ramachandran speculated that laughter and its contagion provide the needed release from the monkeys' collective state of fear, vigilance, and behavioral orientation toward seeking safety. Through laughter, the monkeys can signal that the coast is clear for the troop to return to other sorts of monkey business. Through laughter, the monkeys can indicate that no predator is near and danger has passed. The fact that laughter is contagious also makes sense in this context. Just as fear contagion allows alarm to pass quickly through the troop, so, too, does relief as signaled by laughter contagion. Finally, humor, along with fear, is registered in the same subcortical emotion-detecting structure of the brain, the amygdala.

From a neurobiological point of view, as mentioned previously, laughter, like the cough, hiccup, or retch, is a closed program, with its origins deep in the subcortical roots of the mammalian brain (Panksepp, 1998). Input from the environment and postnatal experiences activate the program but do not shape the circuit, which remains a fixed sequence akin to reflexes or other stereotyped behavior. From a biomechanical point of view, human beings laugh in staccato bursts that are emitted only during exhalations. A wide range from two to around ten "ha-ha" bursts punctuates a single outbreath. Try it to feel this. By contrast, chimps laugh both during the inhalation and exhalation phase of a breath. The one-to-one correspondence between the "hee-hee" linked to each of the chimp's inhalations and exhalations results in a pantlike pattern. Try making this sound as well. Provine (2000) speculated that this difference in laughs between humans and chimps is highly significant. In fact, he hypothesized that it illuminates, if not explains, why humans can use their vocal cords to talk, while monkeys cannot. Because humans have a looser coupling between breathing and vocalizing, they can modulate their exhalations during laughter in just the way necessary for speech. Meanwhile, the tight coupling between breath and laughter in chimps and other primates leaves no wiggle room for the play of air through the vocal cords that is required for speech.

TICKLED PINK

Human infants emit their first true laugh at around 3 or 4 months, a seminal event that occurs in conjunction with the tickle instinct in parents, as was demonstrated in the case of Macy and her baby. The impulse to tickle a baby's belly or toes is an early manifestation of later rough-and-tumble play. This is a universal urge that humans share with chimps, gorillas, and other primates. As part of his investigation of laughter, Provine wondered how the tickle instinct that begins in infancy continues to play itself out

during the life span. So Provine and his undergraduate students conducted a survey by interviewing people of all ages.

Results indicated that interest both in tickling and being tickled is primarily a young person's sport. Respondents younger than 40 years old
were more than 10 times more likely to report having been tickled during
the previous week then those 40 and older, with 43% of younger respondents reporting being tickled versus only 4% of older respondents. According to Provine, this sharp drop-off in the "mammalian triad of tickle, touch
and play" means that older people neither feel very ticklish in their bodies
nor are interested in tickling as an expression of affection, except toward
small babies. As for younger people, incidences of tickling or being tickled
are most likely to occur with intimate others, including relatives, lovers,
and close friends. For teenagers and people in their twenties, tickling is
most connected with courtship rituals. Tickling especially is a handy, nonverbal way to approach a potential romantic partner. In this manner, consensual tickling relates to courtship rituals and sexual foreplay.

Provine noted that the link between tickling and sex seems less specula-
tive when we consider that the Dutch word for clitoris is *kittelaar*, which
means "the organ of being tickled or titillated." After all, tickling involves a
rhythm of reciprocity that necessarily implicates an other. As mentioned, it
is impossible to tickle oneself. And the intensity of the tickle experience
varies inversely with a person's control over and predictability of the touch
stimulus. Provine suggested that the response to a tickle requires a *nonself
detector* in the brain, which signals the presence of an outside influence by
comparing the body's own sense of itself through proprioception with outside stimulation perceived though exteroception. The less predictable the
stimulus, the greater the "nonselfness" or otherness that was perceived.

With babies, during the introduction of otherness through tickling, the
line between pleasure and pain is quite thin. The episode remains pleasurable as long as the tickling event remains consensual. Indeed, an
attuned parent knows when to retreat from touch to allow the baby to recover. Just as the misattuned parent can trigger fussing, crying, and eventual terror in babies through unwanted touch, there is also a connection
between nonconsensual tickling and sadomasochistic sexual rituals (see
Figure 5.8). The use of bondage and feathers to set up tickle torture
blends with other fetishes, such as attraction toward feet or being stepped
on. These fetishes shade into heavier forms of sadomasochistic bondage
and even sexual torture.

Throughout the ages, nonconsensual tickling has also been used as
a form of torture, even to the point of death. Nonconsensual tickling as
torture relates to the potential invasion of personal space by predators.
Ticklishness in all our most sensitive areas—under the armpits, around
our ears, necks, middle torsos, or private parts—evolved as a mechanism
to detect and flick away invading creatures such as bugs, snakes, or scorpi-
ons. Tickling simulates the invasion of larger, perhaps carnivorous, preda-

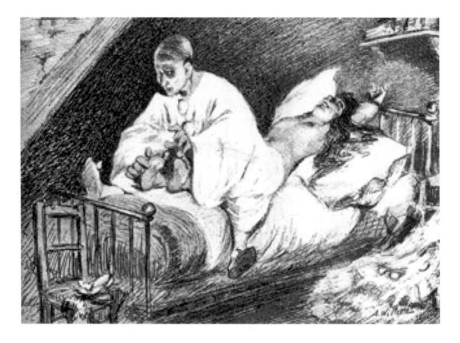

Figure 5.8. In this example of nonconsensual tickling, which is a common form of light sadomasochistic sexuality, Pierrot is tickling Columbine to death in a drawing that appeared on December 7, 1888, in Le Pierrot. (Public domain, Adolphe Willet)

tors in an arena that is safe. And in these origins, we can see, too, how tickling and accompanying laughter relate to the relief and pleasure of false alarm predation.

From this vantage point, my work with Goldie appeared to be an embodiment of the False Alarm Theory as it operates among humans. For 8 years, Goldie had gotten more and more frozen in her body and in her marriage. She was continually in a state of hyperarousal in the presence of her husband where she found it literally, as well as figuratively, difficult to breathe. By conceiving of Jake as capable of extending empathy but withholding it on purpose, this only made her feel worse and more constricted inside. At the point of recognizing that Jake could not help himself, that he had a blind spot that prevented him from extending empathy, she let go of some defensive bracing and released much pent-up emotion. Through the out-breathing of laughter, Goldie found relief and a safe spot on which to stand and reexamine her marriage, however temporary that relief was to her.

From the standpoint of Stephen Porges's polyvagal theory (2011), laughter can seal the deal of release or repair by emerging when the patient moves from a primary stance of defensive fight, flight, or freeze back to the safety of full social engagement. This kind of safety is no small feat, and as clinicians we should recognize the importance of laughter as a signal in this regard.

Perhaps this fundamental safety and relief out of which laughter sometimes emerges connects with the recent social phenomenon of laughter yoga. Put simply, laughter yoga uses laughter in the context of a social group as a complete well-being workout. The brainchild of Dr. Madan Kataria, a physician from Mumbai, India, the first laughter club was launched in 1995, with now over 6,000 social laughter clubs existing in approximately 60 cities (a good example of how to laugh is shown in Figure 5.9).

Combining unconditional laughter with yogic breathing (pranayama), anyone can laugh for no reason. By simulating laughter as a body exercise

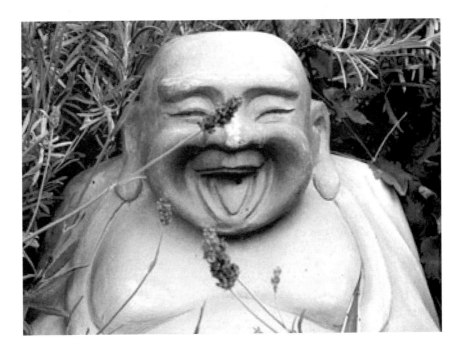

Figure 5.9. The holiness of laughter has universal resonances. The laughing Buddha is an ancient Chinese folklore figure who should not be confused with the historical Buddha, Siddhartha Gautama, the founder of Buddhism. The laughing Buddha is usually depicted as a fat and bald man who carries his scant possessions in a cloth sack. While lacking in material wealth, the laughing Buddha symbolizes happiness, plenitude, and the wisdom of contentment. To rub his belly is believed to bring wealth, good luck, and prosperity. (Public domain, courtesy of Maurizio Jaya Costantino)

by using eye contact and childlike playfulness, social engagement through laughter quickly becomes contagious. Who knows, perhaps social contagion will spread to psychology as well, so that a new school of laughter therapy will arise.

WRAP-UP

Clinical intuition frequently expresses itself in idiosyncratic ways, including our sense of humor. William James asserted that "common sense and a sense of humor are the same thing, moving at different speeds. A sense of humor is just common sense, dancing" (1890). This chapter revealed the many faces of humor within psychotherapy as guided by clinical intuition. Whether initiated by the patient or therapist, humor represents an invitation to communicative play that holds the potential to open up new realms of mutual bonding and exploration. Whereas early chapters asserted clinical intuition to involve implicit processes, this chapter asserted humor within psychotherapy to involve implicit communication about the nature of the therapeutic relationship. Sometimes we collude with patients around defenses and sometimes we bond through direct emotional exchange. In both cases, humor represents an emotionally evocative and expressive form of communication, as intuitively wrought, running alongside the content of our narratives.

Clifton Paul Fadiman suggests, "A sense of humor is the ability to understand a joke—and that joke is oneself." Indeed, some assert that humor in and of itself has healing properties. Norman Cousins (1979) claimed to heal a life-threatening illness through megadoses of Vitamin C along with promoting a positive attitude by watching old movies and laughing uproariously. Cousins started a revolution in patient activism, partly through the use of humor to boost the body's capacity for healing. Research reveals that laughter, joy, and positive emotions generally reduce stress and boost immunity (e.g., Borins, 2003; Miracle, 2007; Snowden, 2003). These positive states help to prevent illness and ease its recovery. Indeed, the whole movement of positive psychology suggests that something very profound exists in the mind/body relationships among enjoyment of life, well-being, and longevity.

Stand-Up for Mental Health, an organization formed in 1995 in Vancouver, Canada, is spearheaded by David Granirer. The members consist of mentally challenged people, some of whom have serious diagnoses, who are trying to laugh their way back to mental health through stand-up comedy centered upon their own conditions. Videos of the members' performances can be seen on YouTube, while a documentary about the training and a comedy road trip is also available for viewing. Perhaps the plight of these noble individuals embodies Irwin Cobb's assertion that "humor is merely tragedy standing on its head with its pants torn" or Groucho Marx's quip that "humor is reason gone mad." The intuitive use of humor for self-reflection can help to ground us, even if we feel lost and have strayed far from our inner vision.

In order to bring home the relevance of this chapter to you and your clinical practice, consider the following:

- Whether young or old, when we gaze at ourselves in the mirror, most of us look at or search for wrinkles on our faces. When gazing at your face in the mirror, what habitual emotion or emotions do the lines indicate? Do your lines speak of sorrow or worry? What about laugh lines? If this is hard to determine, try making exaggerated sad, worried, or gleeful expressions on your face to see which wrinkles get picked up most.
- When was the last time you had a belly laugh? Can you remember? If so, how long ago was the episode? What made you laugh? What about a time you laughed so hard you cried? If you cannot remember, why not?
- Did you laugh often as a child? What did this state of affairs reflect about your childhood? Do you laugh more or less now? Why? How do you feel about this?
- How important is humor to you personally? What about in a mate or close companions?
- What about professionally? Do you cultivate humor consciously in your work with patients? If so, can you remember the last time you laughed deeply with a patient? What was being communicated about the nature of your relationship?
- If you do not cultivate humor consciously, would you like to do so or are you content with your level of seriousness?

Humor is one aspect of creativity that is intuitively expressed and borne of the imagination. The next chapter addresses other aspects of inner vision and imagination as cornerstones in the healing process.

CHAPTER 6

Lighting the Way

You cannot depend on your eyes when your imagination is out of focus.
—Mark Twain

The imagination is a territory. Its fate parallels that of the third world. It is feared, disdained, starved, colonized and co-opted. However, it still retains hidden places, inaccessible heights, unfathomable depths, unmapped territories that remain unindustrialized, uncomputerized, unelectrified but illuminated by natural light, insight, fire, beeswax candles, luciérnagas, and occasional strikes of brilliant lightning in the blood.
—Deena Metzger

THE HUMAN IMAGINATION REPRESENTS THE pinnacle of evolution. Through inner channels of the imagination, we can see through the eyes of others, travel back to the past, anticipate future circumstances, visit imaginary places, and create impossible worlds. As with any inner tool, the imagination can be wielded in service of defense, if retreat into fantasy serves as a refuge from trauma or an escape from reality. Alternatively the imagination can be wielded in service of self-expression and creativity, when it serves as a portal into reality where future possibilities are subsequently manifested.

Psychotherapists use the imagination partly in service of empathy, which is a key ingredient to the healing process. If we do not understand what if feels like to see the world through the eyes of our patients and what it is like to be them, we cannot establish a solid platform through the therapeutic bond. But this kind of present-centered empathy is not enough. When a patient feels like she is drowning emotionally, simply to be understood by her therapist might feel as if someone is drowning alongside her (see Figure 6.1).

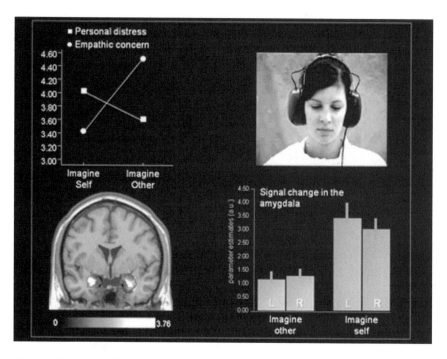

Figure 6.1. As therapists, we must strike a balance between emotional and cognitive aspects of empathy. If therapists resonate too strongly with patients, we can become preoccupied with personal distress. Participants watched video clips of people exposed to painful sounds as part of a medical treatment. Those instructed to imagine how they would feel in a patient's situation revealed a strong increase in blood flow to the amygdala, along with subjective reports of anxiety and personal distress. Participants who were instructed to imagine how the patient felt each had decreased activity in the amygdala, reduced feelings of anxiety, and increased reports of sympathy and concerns for the patient. (Courtesy of Jean Decety)

Along with the capacity to regulate our own emotional distress there is another critical ingredient that is necessary: the capacity to envision a different and better future. Within therapists, this kind of inner vision might arise as a vague hope or sense of patient potential, or it might emerge in the form of specific images that guide us along the therapeutic path. Whatever form such a vision takes, through the imagination not only do we reach into the minds, hearts, and worlds of others, but we also look forward toward the future. Through the imagination, we sense possibilities and open up fields of potential, as if to provide maps to areas of wonder and curiosity. How might we be of service? Where will the openings be? How can we work around those defenses? Where might intuition and creativity align, so that novel solutions become possible?

In this chapter, I discuss how the imagination works hand in hand with clinical intuition. Imagination is the pinnacle of the "high right" brain devoted to processing and producing novelty. The implicit, intuitive flows of psychotherapy involve dynamic arcs that encompass the past, present, and future. The relational unconscious is an imaginary realm where the bodies, brains, and full psyches of the patient and therapist become intertwined beneath the level of awareness. Within the relational unconscious, various temporal flows of bodily, brain, and mental processes coexist, each operating on a different timescale.

Within the affective core of the therapeutic process, the therapist's ability to remain regulated in counterpoint and contrast with the dysregulated emotion of patients requires the imaginative capacity to hold open possibilities for a better future, even while immersed in intolerable states. Within a complexity model of mental health (Marks-Tarlow, 2008a; Siegel, 1999), the widest capacity for fluidity, variability, and adaptability requires an open future not tethered to the past. Ultimately, it is not just therapists but also patients who must envision possibilities for change in order to fully embody new ways to be, see the world, and relate to others (see Figure 6.2).

This chapter explores how psychotherapists and patients intuitively draw on visual imagery and other forms of sensory-based imagination. Imagination promotes patient self-expression while assisting therapists to intuit a path through psychotherapy. I begin with a case study of a man named George and my efforts to help him deepen into his body's primary affective experience. George produced spontaneous imagery that became a fulcrum for subsequent work. George's image served as a central metaphor that pointed backward and forward at the same time. I next examine the neurobiological sources of imagination within neural processes of the brain and within embodied metaphor. Not only was George's imagery a beautiful representation of his early implicit relational experience, but it also informed his current struggles with others, including with me, within transference and countertransference dynamics.

The beauty of imagination is its capacity to embrace the whole of things. George's imagery illuminated the central problem as it already existed, as well as what the future might hold. George's main dilemma—how to recapture freedom to feel fully and manifest dreams creatively—has universal resonances. In its healthiest manifestation, whether in the therapist or patient, imagination inspires vitality through fuller self-expression.

WHEN FEELINGS BUBBLE UP

When George was a boy, he loved to play Dungeons and Dragons. But then he hit adolescence, and he put the game away, suppressing what he feared

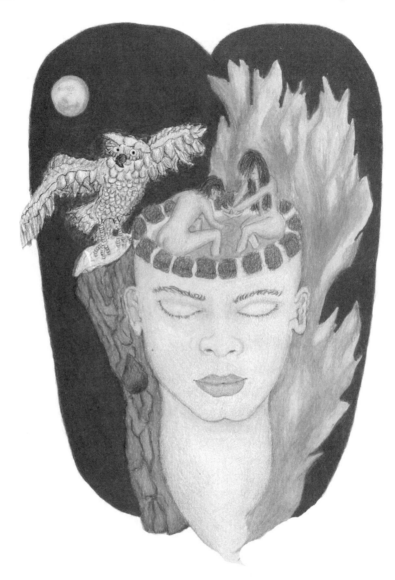

Figure 6.2. Within psychotherapy, intuition and imagination go hand in hand. Although therapists may descend into the depths of despair, helplessness, and pain at times, we recharge and rebalance through reconnecting to flames of our own passions and depths of our inspiration. As a therapist, I believe one of my strengths is the continual capacity to make meaning out of tragedy combined with an almost endless fountain of hope and imagination for a better life to come. (Courtesy of the author)

were "nerdy" urges in hopes of "looking cool" instead. George is a likable, high-functioning guy. Yet despite his strong relationships, meaningful work, and a host of other strengths, George's life is partly a cautionary tale about creativity—once forsaken, creativity is easily forsaken again. George entered film school with every intention to write screenplays, yet his creative dreams were waylaid by an internship that he had skillfully leveraged into a stable job. George was too tempted to work on the production side, with its steady employment and good salary, than to risk the life of a poor, failed artist. Although grateful for his job George secretly envied the writers with whom he came into daily contact. Once in a while George would take a stab at his own creative writing, but like the Dungeons and Dragons games so many years earlier, the writing fragments wound up folded up or tucked away in books, never cohering into a finished product.

George was a relative newlywed who entered therapy at the encouragement of his wife, Sue, due to her discord with George's mother. In this classic scenario, Sue and her mother-in-law struggled to redraw family lines. George's mother wanted the couple to spend every free moment with her. Sue wanted George to spend more time with her parents. George, who considered himself an easygoing guy and perennial peacemaker, just wanted everyone to get along. George entered therapy feeling a lot of pressure, especially from his wife. Sue was pressing George to confront his mother, and this left him feeling rather frantic.

"No one stands up to my mother!" George declared, giving me a darting glance, as if checking to see if I really understood this behemoth task. "She has *really strong feelings* and is *very* quick to feel slighted and hurt. She is normally so nice, caring, and attentive. But *all of it* has to be on her terms. In our family she *always* gets her way. *Everybody* caters to her, including my father. Now I've gone and married someone who also has strong feelings. I feel caught. I'm trapped in the middle of these two. And I really don't like it here. I just want everybody to calm down."

I said, "I can see your discomfort in the pained expression on your face. Your dilemma seems particularly hard when both women are so articulate and expressive. But I have to tell you something—and this is just a gut reaction on my part. When you said just now that *all* you want is for everybody to calm down, this is hard for me to believe. My intuition says there's more going on than that. I'm guessing there is more to your perspective— a whole set of feelings about each issue you mention—whom to visit, when to go, under what circumstances. But it may be too hard for you to hear your own voice in the midst of such loud feelings expressed by the others."

As George thought about my comment, his expression changed in a way that was riveting. His face shifted in a most unusual way—in opposite directions. This was not the vertical kind of split we see when, for example, the left side of a person's mouth descends into a sneer, while the right side creeps up into a smile. That is what happens when the socially acceptable, public right side of the face conceals private emotions that are more evident on the left side of the face. This was quite different, for George's face was split horizontally, such that the top and bottom halves expressed completely different emotions. George's eyes welled up with tears that spilled into a steady stream down his face; meanwhile, his mouth broke into a smile that gathered force into laughter.

"Wow, you are crying and laughing at the same time!? What is your inner experience?"

"I didn't realize until you said it that I might actually have feelings and opinions about all of these things as well. I had been too busy fielding everybody else's emotions."

"How does that realization leave your body feeling?" I asked, wanting to stick with the affective core of things.

"I'm not sure. . . ."

"Would you like to close your eyes for a minute, to see if you can sink into it?"

George closed his eyes, growing still. After a few seconds, from somewhere deep inside came a tiny, gravelly voice trying to eke its way out from a catch in the middle of George's throat: "I see myself floating in a bubble. I can see through the walls. They are clear but very thick. Everything inside the bubble is muted. My words can't get out. Neither can I."

As George opened his eyes, he blinked a couple of times, sitting silently, waiting for my response.

"Your bubble image captures a poignant dilemma. I can see why you're sad about being so insulated and emotionally suppressed, and I imagine you're also relieved at feeling understood and understanding the problem more fully yourself."

"Exactly!" George replied, amidst more tears and laughter.

EMBODIED MEANING

The cognitive linguists George Lakoff and Mark Johnson (1980, 1999) asserted that *all cognitive activity is embodied,* because it derives from a primary set of metaphors that surround how the body moves, functions, and interacts in the physical and social world in which we are embedded. The psychoanalyst Arnold Modell (2003) has picked up on the relevance of Lakoff and Johnson's work for psychotherapy by writing extensively on how the body uses metaphor to bridge disconnected experience, create somatic templates, and weave the illusion of constancy during continual change. George's image of being in a bubble was an embodied metaphor. The image was embodied literally, because George pictured his entire body encased within the bubble (see Figure 6.3). The image was also embodied figuratively, as George's core affective and bodily experience became a source point for his imagination.

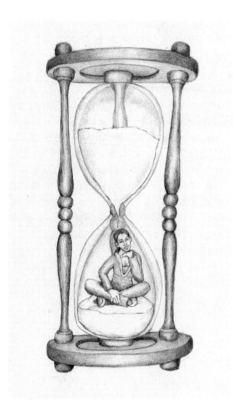

Figure 6.3. One reason that metaphor is so powerful during psychotherapy is the same reason that it's so powerful in art. Metaphor speaks to the heart of our emotions quite loudly. George envisioned himself to be trapped in a soap bubble, but there are many ways to stretch this metaphor. In this drawing, a girl trapped in an hourglass depicts the dangers of technology backfiring, if we become trapped by the very devices we create to save time. (Courtesy of the author)

Here are some previous thoughts about the importance of metaphors within psychotherapy:

Derived initially from our most concrete interactions with others and the world, the body employs metaphor as a kind of "corporeal imagination," to use Cornelius Castorius' phrase, for transferring experience from inside to outside, past to present, one sensory mode to another. Within psychotherapy this preverbal aspect has been called the "unthought known" by Christopher Bollas (1987) and more recently "the unrepressed unconscious" by Mauro Mancia (2006). . . . By fusing various perceptual, emotion, and cognitive capacities, metaphor-making becomes a primary way to construct meaning. Through metaphor, we interpret and transform experience; mark value; declare relationship; and hold mirrors up to our being, doing and moving in the world. By welding discrete experiences together, metaphor expresses a sense of continuity versus fragmentation of the self through time. (Marks-Tarlow, 2008a, p. 93)

Verticality and balance are among Lakoff and Johnson's primary metaphors. This makes a great deal of sense given the early developmental milestones of human beings. Babies universally shift from the horizontal posture of lying down to more vertical postures by first rolling over, then sitting upright, then crawling, and eventually rising up to balance and walk on two legs. Each shift is associated with increased mobility, agency, and potency in the world. This near universal sequence is likely a prime factor in our culture's association of the direction of up with good things and the direction of down with bad things.

On the positive side:

"She's sitting *on top of the world*."

"Give me *a high five*."

"*Thumbs up* for that!"

"His prospects are *looking up*."

On the negative side:

"He's feeling *under the weather*."

"Her fortune took a *downturn*."

"What a *lowlife!*"

"Never do business *under the table*."

During psychotherapy we intuitively choose our language by tapping into the deep connections between words and their bodily, affective, and relational resonances. Whether expressed through concrete gestures or abstract words, these associations have deep roots that are automatic and implicit. The importance of verticality and balance relates as much to our species' history as it does to our personal one, harkening back to a point when Homo sapiens diverged from our primate ancestors in order to walk stably and consistently on two feet. At that seminal bifurcation in evolution, our arms and hands were freed for tool making, care giving, and other tasks related to increasingly complex social and cultural contexts.

BALANCE THROUGHOUT THE LIFESPAN

Between the ages of 9 months to 1 year, each baby replicates the species' trend from moving on all fours to balancing vertically on two feet—a particularly thrilling event for parents. Over time we easily take for granted our capacities to retain balance and a vertical stance. Yet the importance of these issues does not stop in early childhood. Verticality and balance return as physical challenges if we imbibe too much alcohol or ingest too many drugs or suffer from various neurological conditions. Yet for most of us, as we develop both physically and cognitively, issues of verticality and balance take on increasingly metaphorical dimensions, as when we strive toward *high ideals* while retaining a *balanced outlook* on life. To achieve wisdom is to achieve the *height* of complex and useful under-standing about life and other *lofty* subjects (the subject of Chapter 8).

In order to illustrate the importance of verticality and balance as cen-tral metaphors at other critical points of life, I next tell a story about my brother, John Marks. The year was 1980, a time in my brother's life when he was highly off balance, metaphorically speaking. John was in between everything—waffling, alone, and unsure of his next steps. His then wife had just left their marriage. He was midway through a yearlong teaching engagement at Harvard University, in a position based more on past ac-complishments than on future directions. John had just written two books that brought him notoriety. The first, *The CIA and the Cult of Intel-ligence*, cowritten with Victor Marchetti (1974), exposed the CIA's clan-destine operations abroad. John's second book, *The Search for the Manchurian Candidate* (1979) uncovered the CIA's mind control at-tempts through the agency's covert experimentation with LSD, hypnosis, personality assessment, and other behavior science techniques—using unwitting test subjects, prostitutes, and the criminally insane. While my brother had taken tremendous risks up until this point and these risks had paid off, he had also effectively burned many of his professional bridges. John was left bereft, with little clue of where to go next.

During this period of pain and confusion and for no apparent reason, one day John dropped to the floor unconscious. He could not be roused and was taken to the hospital. The rest of the family—my mother, father, sister, and me—rushed to Boston. My mother and sister were beside themselves, because of the history of a similar traumatic event in the fam-ily. Many years before, my mother's father had contracted viral meningitis. He, too, had fallen into a coma and lay unconscious in a bed for an entire year. During that year, my mother's mother had died from a heart attack from all the stress. At the end of a year, my grandfather inexplicably and miraculously awoke to regain his full mental capacities, a new chance at life, and even a new wife at the ripe age of 72.

Maybe because I am much younger than my siblings and was not alive when all of this unfolded, I felt clearheaded during my brother's emergency and sent everybody else home. I stayed on in Boston alone at my brother's bedside to serve as the advocate and conduit for his friends and colleagues. Meanwhile the doctors tried to figure out what was going on medically. After a week, John was diagnosed with a subdural hematoma. A surgeon immediately drilled two holes into my brother's skull in order to relieve the internal pressure, and he subsequently added two more such holes. As if by magic, after more than 2 weeks, John awakened from his coma.

Not long after recovering from this medical incident, John founded Search for Common Ground in 1982 (see www.sfcg.org). Today, Search is the world's largest, nongovernmental organization for conflict prevention and resolution, and it helps communities and whole countries to transform ethnic and other forms of social and political conflict into cooperative action. Rather than working only "top down" with vertical, hierarchical governmental agencies, Search also works "bottom up" with everyday people, largely through the horizontal spread afforded by the arts, sports, educational systems, television shows, and radio programming. In both a literal and metaphorical sense, John's "fall" in life eventually helped him to regain balance and a new vertical position. In the process, he not only transformed himself, but he also has helped significant portions of the world at large.

When I recently told my brother I was writing a book about clinical intuition, his ears perked up. He invited me, along with his current wife and professional partner, Susan Collin Marks, to a powwow to talk about his ideas about intuition, creativity, and social entrepreneurship. Much to my surprise, John conceptualized his style of running Search to revolve around intuition. He and Susan face most conflict resolution encounters with years of organizational and personal experience, but without any fixed plan of action. This stance positions them to be sensitively attuned as they feel their way through different peoples, cultures, conflicts, and countries.

We were all struck by parallels between this strategy for conflict transformation and clinical encounters. My brother and Susan have formalized their approach by developing 13 maxims for social entrepreneurship:

- Start from vision.
- Be an applied visionary.
- Be prepared to deal with high levels of complexity.
- *"On s'engage; puis on voit."* [This is a quote from Napoleon that means "one becomes engaged, and then one sees the possibilities."]
- Practice aikido.
- Make "yes-able" propositions.
- Enroll credible supporters.
- Apply *fingerspitzengefühl* [a German word for having an intuitive sense of knowing at the tip of your finger].
- Demonstrate chutzpah.
- Develop good metaphors and models.
- Have a high tolerance for ambiguity.
- Find trimtab points. [On ships and airplanes, the trimtab is a tiny rudder at the leverage point and it can turn the craft with a minimum of effort.]
- Be persistent. (Marks & Collin Marks, 2009)

Clearly, each principle relates to an intuitive style of program development and conflict transformation. Each principle also relates to the intuitive side of our work as psychotherapists. During this lunch John introduced me to the wonderful German word *fingerspitzengefühl*, which, as mentioned above, translates literally as "knowledge felt at the tip of a finger." When John gives talks, he mentions this word often. To my brother, the word *fingerspitzengefühl* carries the power to legitimize what otherwise might seem like a vague concept and process. By giving something a name and putting it into words, suddenly it springs to life—an embodied metaphor indeed!

THE POWER OF METAPHOR

Daniel Stern understood the power of metaphor within therapy by stating, "When psychopathology is viewed from the clinical point of view, the primary task is to find the narrative point of origin—invariably, the key metaphor(s)" (1985, p. 282). When he wrote this line, Stern wanted to highlight a difference between the neuroses and Axis II character disorders. In the neuroses, a single traumatic event can serve as the *actual* point of origin for symptoms. When the real origin of psychopathology is this obvious, metaphor becomes unnecessary. Yet, as I have written previously (Marks-Tarlow, 2008a), even here metaphor can be useful. *Psyche's Veil* details the treatment of a patient who developed a simple trauma after awakening in great fear during a major earthquake. He was on the upper floor of a hotel, in the dark, and in unfamiliar surroundings. Subsequent to this event, this man's fear of becoming trapped evolved into his fear of leaving the safety of his home. Within psychotherapy, my patient made great progress at the point when we treated the early morning earthquake as a metaphorical *wake-up call* for self-examination. This included switching the search for safety from outer to inner sources.

By contrast to cases with clearly identifiable traumatic origins, in cases of character disorder, pathology tends to be borne out of repetitive interactional patterns. Developing slowly and cumulatively, these conditions start during infancy, beginning before episodic memory (Schore, 2001), such that no actual point of origin exists. In Stern's words, "The insult (or pattern) is effectively present and acting at all developmental points." Indeed, a host of data have linked disorganized, insecure attachment borne from early physical, sexual, or emotional abuse and neglect with later posttraumatic conditions, including borderline personality disorder (e.g., Weaver & Clum, 1993). Research tools such as the Strange Situation reveal that episodes of severe distress that last as short as 15 seconds can predict severe psychopathology years later.

In this sort of pattern it becomes impossible to pinpoint the precise source of a trauma. There are simply too many incidents. Here, it helps to heed Stern's words. To seek a narrative point of origin through metaphor is to connect imagery and other sensory modalities directly with affectively loaded experience. As a brief clinical example, in response to not understanding a comment of mine, a patient recalled sitting at the dinner table with the rest of the family as a little girl. Everyone was speaking French; the girl's failure to understand the language left her feeling ashamed, lonely, and disconnected. The imagery of the little girl at the dinner table with French-speaking adults is a powerful metaphor that could be used repeatedly during psychotherapy. In this way, metaphors serve as a heuristic that allows therapists and patients alike to compare earlier states of mind with present ones.

Whereas people with the Axis II disorders often suffer severe symptoms and limitations, George was successful in love and work but lacked a formal diagnosis. Nonetheless, when conducting psychotherapy with high-functioning patients, the use of metaphor helps to access subtle, inner landscapes that stem from preverbal roots. On the surface, George's life was rich and filled with meaningful relationships and activities. So it took some time, trust, and finesse to sink down into subcortical zones where George's issues revolved around the *absence of strong feeling*. To tap into George's spontaneous imagery was to find a vehicle into suppressed aspects of the self borne of subtle relational dynamics. Like dreams that emerge from the relational unconscious to prompt, poke, or provoke the analyst (Sands, 2011), George's metaphor of being encased in a bubble was an act of imagination both stimulated by and in turn stimulating to its relational context.

The use of metaphor during psychotherapy can help the patient to launch his or her creative imagination, identified since antiquity as a primary tool for emotional and mind/body healing (see Pincus & Sheikh, 2009). As part of my deep belief that clinical work, when most effective, is an inherently and intersubjectively creative enterprise, I have suggested that "within psychotherapy, complexity is revealed partly by the metaphors we choose. . . . The art and science of psychotherapy merge within its metaphors. Like liquid poetry that congeals into precise methods of inquiry, metaphors frame how we look with patients and ultimately what we find" (Marks-Tarlow, 2008a, p. 92).

Arnold Modell argued that imagination is central to the creation of meaning. Drawing on diverse fields—from philosophy to neurobiology—Modell assigned imagination a key role in linking past relational memory with present circumstances and possible futures. Modell cited Giambattista Vico, born in 1668, as an early figure who understood *meaning as embodied imaginatively through our total affective interest in the world and in others.* Vico's insight has been confirmed by neurobiological evidence for the simulation model of empathy, by which we understand others first by simulating their emotions, intentions, and actions internally as the basis for our imaginative capacity to recreate their inner and outer worlds (Goldman, 2008). Modell speculated that, during evolution, acquisition of the cognitive capacity for metaphoric thought emerged out of imaginative bases that originated both before the human capacity for language and were quite separate from it.

EMBODIED METAPHOR

Modell's perspective dovetails with that of the British psychiatrist Iain McGilchrist (2009). McGilchrist cited ample evidence that metaphorical thought is a specialty of the right brain, with roots in music, the emotions, and the body. McGilchrist presented a picture of the two cerebral hemispheres as "opponent processors": As the perspective of one hemisphere comes to the forefront to dominate conscious awareness, the perspective of the other gets inhibited and fades into the background. As with other opponent processes, such as color perception, this enables exquisitely fine modulation: "It is neither that the products of one hemisphere negate the products of the other, nor that in some bland sense they merely 'complement' one another. Their incompatibility permits instead, in a dialectical synthesis, something new to arise" (McGilchrist, 2009, p. 91).

According to McGilchrist, the left hemisphere operates independently of its context by narrowing focus, pinpointing ideas, and manipulating concepts according to internal, linear logic. The left hemisphere shaves away all irrelevancies in order to isolate essential facts and rescue bare abstractions from their relativity of context. By contrast, McGilchrist described the right hemisphere as thriving in ambiguity while embracing the novelty of the moment through the details of context. The realm of the right includes the messiness of the body, with its multimodal affective, sensory, and motor signals. This helps the right to make perceptual links between words as well as bind emotional truths through wide expanses of vision and open frontiers of imagination.

McGilchrist also linked metaphor with the primacy of implicit over explicit processes:

> Metaphor (subserved by the right hemisphere) comes *before* denotation (subserved by the left). This is both a historical and an epistemological truth. Metaphorical meaning is in every sense prior to abstraction and explicitness. The very words tell one this: one cannot draw something away (Latin, *abs-* away, *trahere* pull), unless there is something to draw it away from. One cannot unfold something and make it explicit (Latin, *ex-* out, *plicare* fold), unless it is already folded. The roots of explicitness lie in the implicit. As Lichtenberg said, "Most of our expressions are metaphorical—the philosophy of our forefathers lies hidden in them." (p. 179)

Because the right hemisphere takes what is said within its entire context, it is particularly adept at weighing similarities and differences in order to produce and process novel metaphorical expressions, which is so important to self-discovery during psychotherapy. Whereas familiar phrases activate the left hemisphere, unfamiliar ones activate the right hemisphere. Once a phrase, even a metaphorical one, has become old or clichéd, it will move into the left-side processing. The work of Pobric, Mashal, Faust, and Lavidor (2008) indicated that it is the specific combination of novelty with the metaphorical bringing together of disparate ideas that implicates the right hemisphere. This division of labor conforms to recent speculation (MacNeilage, Rogers, & Vallortigara, 2009) about the origins of lateralization, or differences between the left and right brains, of early vertebrates dating back half a billion years. Whereas the left brain specialized in habitual tasks, like hunting or eating, the right was reserved for novel tasks, like perceiving strangers or danger.

Imagination is a potent tool for change (see Figure 6.4). Research in the area of neuroplasticity confirms the integration of imagination with embodied action. Using transcranial magnetic stimulation, researchers have repeatedly shown in rats, monkeys, and humans that *imagining* an action or a physical task (e.g., piano playing) enables one to *perform* it, at times as efficiently and accurately as someone who actually practiced it. The brain physically changes as we are rehearsing or imagining, and this can be tracked (Doidge, 2007).

Along with embodied action, metaphor also exists within embodied experience more broadly. In an interesting article in the *New York Times* entitled "This Is Your Brain on Metaphors," Robert Sapolsky (2010) identified various subcortical limbic structures as sources for metaphor. For example, much as the neurons of the insula activate when an animal eats a disgusting piece of rotten, fetid food, so, too, do they activate when we feel disgust in other ways (see Figure 6.5):

> Now read in the newspaper about a saintly old widow who had her home foreclosed by a sleazy mortgage company, her medical insurance canceled on flimsy grounds, and got a lousy, exploitative offer at the pawn shop where she tried to hock her kidney dialysis machine. You sit there thinking, those bastards, those people are scum, they're worse than maggots, they make me want to puke . . . and your insula activates.

Another limbic structure that cannot tell the difference between the literal pain of a stubbed toe and the metaphorical pain of a snubbed social encounter is the cingulate cortex within the frontal cerebral lobes (see Figure 6.6). Sapolsky concluded that the brain frequently confuses literal with metaphorical concepts, the real with the symbolic, because evolution is "a tinkerer and not an inventor, and has duct-taped metaphors and symbols to whichever pre-existing brain areas provided the closest fit."

The developmental perspective of Allan Schore views imagery, symbolic thought, and the visual imagination, all so prevalent in metaphor, to represent the apex of "high right" functioning. Most recently, he identified

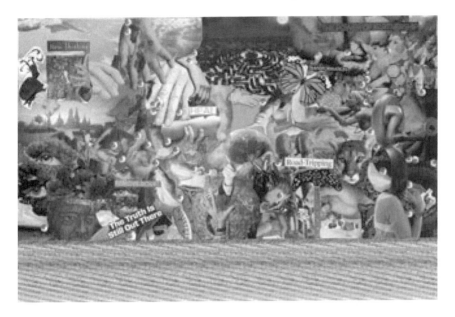

Figure 6.4. The intention board is a wonderful clinical technique for envisioning the future. To leaf through images and intuitively select those that resonate helps to integrate the visual, imaginative modes of the right brain with the analytic skills of the left brain. (Courtesy of Lesleigh Gasbarre)

components of intuition as imagistic cognition and unconscious pattern recognition, including interactional attachment patterns, allocated primarily in the right brain (Schore, 2011).

Whereas Schore emphasized the importance of the therapist discovering the subjective experience of insight in the right emotional and relational brain, Hershberg highlighted the importance of integrating left brain analytic cognitive processing:

> In Schore's model, while the limbic system communicates directly with the right hemisphere, there is a bidirectional flow between the right hemisphere and the left hemisphere, and no direct connection between the left hemisphere and the limbic system emphasizing the crucial importance of and interaction with right hemispheric processes. Fosshage speaks to the fluid interplay of right imagistic symbolic processing and left brain processes at an implicit (subliminal) level. Intuitive hunches emerge out of implicit processes becoming conscious. Bucci would invoke subsymbolic processing as more relevant to the experience of intuition, or a hunch. From my perspective, following Modell (2003), I propose that metaphor formation to be a

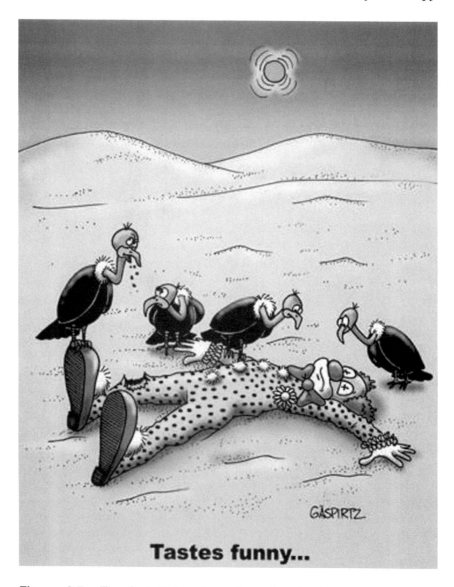

Tastes funny...

Figure 6.5. The fact that rotten, disgusting food co-opts the same subcortical brain area as social disgust—the insula—makes this cartoon all the more funny, if not distasteful. (Courtesy of Oliver Gaspirtz)

bridging implicit/explicit cognitive linguistic concept. Metaphors are imagistically generated from multimodal bodily sensations that both shift meanings between disparate arenas and by means of innovative rearrangements can transform and spawn new perceptions (2011, p. 106).

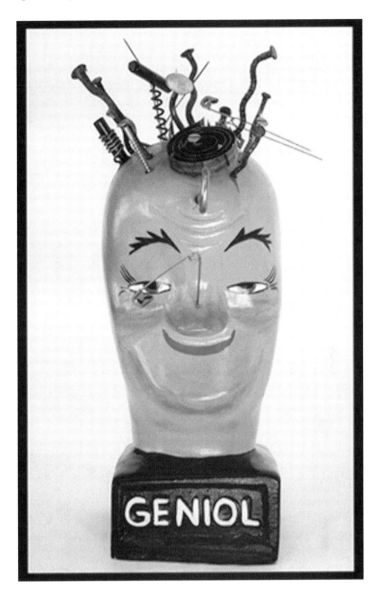

Figure 6.6. Here is a visual metaphor embodied in a literal way. Thanks to Geniol aspirin, the smiling face of a peladito supports the nails, pins, hooks, a corkscrew, and other sharp objects that have been stashed inside his head. The sculptor Jon Hurd was inspired by the famous artist Lucien-Achille Mauzan in order to communicate an image of pain by means of this concrete metaphor for a headache. (Courtesy of Jon Hurd)

STREAMS OF SELF-EXPERIENCE

The word "metaphor" derives from the Greek word *meta*, which means "across," and "pherein," which means "to carry." Whether in speech or in psychotherapy, we use metaphor to transfer or carry meaning over from one domain to another. Modell defined metaphor in line with cognitive linguistics "as a mapping or transfer of meaning between dissimilar domains (from a source domain to a target domain)." (2003, p. 27)

In George's case, I suggest that an understanding of metaphor helped to transfer meaning from past to present circumstances. George's image of being entrapped within a clear bubble, through which he could see perfectly yet could not be heard, seemed to capture the overall feeling of George's early implicit memory of a self that went unseen and who instead had to shape his sense of self around the other. I envision a tiny baby that used his sensitivities to conform to his mother's emotional needs from the start, stifling his awareness of his own feelings and needs in the process. While this can be the formulation for severe pathology, I believe George's mother was dedicated to being the ideal mother, such that her "misses" in attunement were more like blunted blows than sharp whacks.

Specifically, from birth, through an amygdala especially tuned to fearful expressions, this baby appeared to develop a visual hypervigilance to emotional nuance as expressed in the tiny muscles of his mother's face. As George developed, and higher-order regulatory structures like the anterior cingulate and ortibofrontal cortices became available, this baby began to link visual signals to inhibitory impulses so as to dampen down his own emotional experiences and responses. Drawing on the neural circuitry of emotional suppression as described by Alan Fogel (2009), including interoceptive brain structures of the insula, medial frontal lobes, and anterior cingulate, George learned how to conform to his mother's implicit emotional and relational needs, including responding in ways that minimized chances for further emotional triggering effects.

One of the tasks of early childhood is to integrate different streams of exteroceptive sensory information along with interoceptive signals from the insula, limbic structures, and autonomic nervous system about the state of one's own body. Any trauma to the developing baby will reduce the complexity of the mind/body/brain system and affect this capacity for neural integration (Siegel, 2001). With George, complexity became reduced when the visual stream from the eyes served consistently as a channel for inhibition rather than a conduit for the expression of emotion.

A recent family event told of the importance of the visual stream for George's mother. Despite all four of George's siblings now being grown up, his mother still insisted that they carry out the same family tradition dating back to when the children were all young. Each year on Christmas morning, George and his brothers and sisters would come downstairs in their pajamas, in order to receive a gift of a festive cap, knitted scarf, or other holiday garment that George's mother had beautifully crafted during the year. Once everyone was fully decked out, they all then gathered in close for a group photo taken and kept as a memento. Despite feeling foolish carrying out this tradition now, George and Sue continued to do so in deference to George's mother. Recently George felt some agony as he imagined arriving for Christmas in the near but indefinite future with a baby of his own. On the one hand, he could not bear to be the first to break the family tradition; on the other hand, George struggled equally with the image of himself as a parent forced into the childlike stance of parading around in decorative PJs. George's bubble metaphor juxtaposed this very same combination of visual transparency next to aural silence.

In his discussion of originating metaphor, Stern (1985) pointed out how different streams of self-experience carry different affective loadings. "The affective component of the key experience usually resides primarily in one domain of relatedness (that is, in one sense of the self)" (p. 263). The fact that different senses of the self accompany different memories, affective loadings, and even different relationships means that these strands of experience can lie side by side in a way that is not yet fully integrated. Part of the utility of metaphors is that they serve as a vehicle for blending separate channels of the senses.

THE MAN WHO TASTED SHAPES

Not long ago, as I drove my 15-year-old son, Cody, to high school, he told me a story from the day before. Upon finishing, he asked, "Do you see what I'm saying?" "Huh?" I said. "Do you see what I'm saying?" he repeated. "No," I said. "How can I see with my eyes the words that flow invisibly from your mouth? I can only see in space and hear in time."

While using a highly concrete thought to give my son a hard time for a metaphor he unwittingly chose, simultaneously I was having an epiphany. I realized that Cody's rather ordinary expression could only work because the imagination is able to fuse senses of sight and sound into the deeper, more abstract realm of understanding and meaning. We do not have to look far to find the variety of cross-modal expressions sprinkled throughout speech: *loud shirt, bitter wind, sharp cheese, hot babe, flat soda,* and so on.

Synesthesia is the technical word for a literal blending of sensory channels. My son's expression was an everyday, metaphorical example. In the past several years synesthesia has reached above the radar of several prominent neurologists. *The Man Who Tasted Shape* is a book about synesthesia written by Richard Cytowic (1993), a pioneer neurologist and researcher in this area. Only about 10 in a million "suffer" from the neurological condition of literally perceiving "salty visions, purple odors, square tastes, and green wavy symphonies." Yet this realm is filled with many creative geniuses as well. Vladimir Nabokov, David Hockney, Jean Sibelius, Duke Ellington, and Leonard Bernstein have all been identified as synesthetes. Consider these words of the contemporary singer, songwriter, and pianist Tori Amos as written in her recent autobiography: "The song appears as light filament once I've cracked it. As long as I've been doing this, which is more than thirty-five years, I've never seen a duplicate song structure. I've never seen the same light creature in my life. Obviously similar chord progressions follow similar light patterns, but try to imagine the best kaleidoscope ever" (2006, p. 107).

Cytowic considered these true synesthetes as *cognitive fossils* who reveal how all human minds function. Cytowic's journey to understand the evolution of this condition began with clues in the ancient words of Aristotle.

> Each sense discriminates the specific differences of the objects proper to it. Thus sight discriminates between white and black, taste between sweet and bitter, and so on. But we can also discriminate between white and sweet. . . How do we perceive generic differences? It is not possible to discriminate between white and sweet by a difference sense for each of them; there must be one sense to which both of the compared qualities are discernibly present. (2003, p. 86)

Cytowic speculated that all humans are born with senses fused in synesthetic fashion at the subcortical, limbic level, with conscious awareness of this state only reaching a handful of people. Cytowic located synesthesia in the left hippocampus, which functions as a multisensory gateway between the outside world and the rest of the brain. Normal development entails a differentiating out of sensory streams, which are reintegrated at higher levels of brain processing. Ramachandran (2011) disagreed with this theory, believing instead that synesthesia emerges from incomplete pruning between adjacent, initially overlapping sensory processing areas. Incomplete pruning results in the cross-activation of circuitry, as when numbers are perceived as colors due to their close proximity in the fusiform gyrus and near the angular gyrus.

Whatever its origins, synesthesia involves implicit processes that are both automatic and involuntary. Like cross-modal metaphor, synesthesia allows different channels of experience to cross-fertilize one another in ways that facilitate creativity. Many autistic savants draw on synesthesia for their intuitive gifts.

By seeing numbers laid out in spatial dimensions, mathematical savants know the answers to complex calculations automatically and easily, simply by finding them within the landscape. By experiencing musical notes and scales as hues of colors, musical synesthetes enjoy a kaleidoscope of visual images when listening to music (such an experience is usually reserved for people who imbibe hallucinogens) (see Figure 6.7).

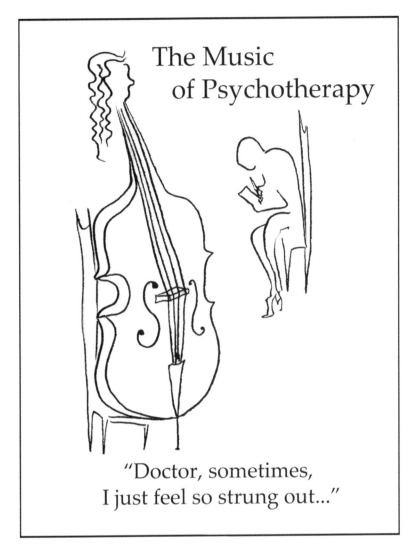

Figure 6.7. Here is an illustration of the music of psychotherapy. Prosody refers to the capacity to read the emotional melody under the musical quality of the words. Babies understand prosody from the start of life, and so they naturally fuse the elements of emotion, music, and words. Clinical intuition is implicitly guided by this kind of synesthetic blend as well. To make this drawing, I borrowed my 13-year-old daughter's cello to model the patient. What she later pointed out to me was my hidden inclusion of the cello's bow as well in the back of the therapist's chair. How fitting that, when writing about imagination as the highest form of intuition, my own imagination proved the point. (Courtesy of the author)

Gus, the patient I introduced in Chapter 2, experienced a kind of musi-cal synesthesia. He was able to enter his music like a landscape, in which he could get lost and shed his separate sense of self while experiencing different dimensions of a song as if within a visual landscape. He could see the space between the notes as well as the junctions where different parts of a piece bump up against one another. Gus's capacity for full im-mersion in his music helped him know what was "right" in a musical com-position without any words or thoughts. He could just see where compo-nents of the piece quite literally needed to go.

Interestingly, Gus perceived his music as emanating from his female side. What is more, Gus discovered a relationship between the music he composed and the emotions he possessed. As our therapy progressed, Gus gained more and more access to his musical side, which had been dormant for years and only accessible with the assistance of marijuana be-fore that. As Gus gained more access to his music, he began to use these synesthetic experiences of full immersion as a road map toward underly-ing emotional experience he could not access from the male side of his identity. The music thus served not only as a road toward self-expression, but it also served as a conduit for self-integration. Although Gus began psychotherapy by hating his female side and asking my help in eliminating her, Gus wound up loving her richness, creativity, and emotional breadth. I return to Gus's case in the chapter on wisdom.

TRANSFORMING THE SELF
THROUGH METAPHOR

Whereas synesthesia works by highlighting the overlap or similarities be-tween two senses, metaphor works by comparing and contrasting both similarities and differences. Modell emphasized the creative potential of metaphor by asserting, "Metaphor not only *transfers* meaning between different domains, but by means of novel recombinations metaphor can *transform* meaning and generate new perceptions. Imagination could not exist without this recombinatory metaphoric process" (2003, p. 27).

I believe the potential within psychotherapy for central metaphors to morph creatively in service of imagination and integration is a key aspect of clinical intuition (see Figure 6.8). I would like to illustrate this in a later iteration of the bubble imagery in my work with George. As the oldest of five children and the only one who was married, George, along with his wife, Sue, continually needed to break new ground with George's par-ents, who loved to run a tight family ship with everyone on board for all occasions. Sue was also close to her parents, who lived nearby. This al-lowed more frequent visits, yet Sue understandably wanted holiday time with her mother and father as well.

One day George received an email from his mother detailing an ex-tended trip to South Africa from February through May being planned by

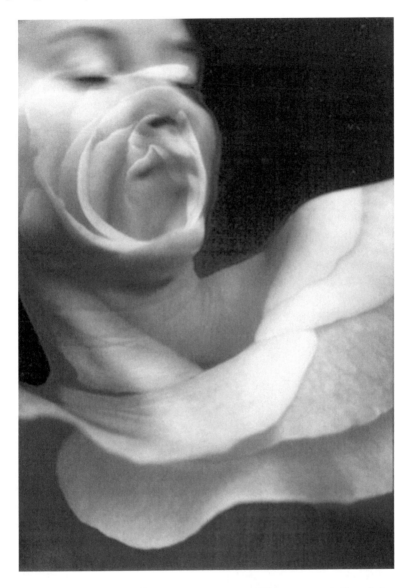

Figure 6.8. In psychotherapy, many practitioners and theorists are illuminating a paradigm shift from thought to emotion and from technique to relationship at the heart of healing. One implication of this is a shift away from doing as a key ingredient to being, that is, how we are with patients may be more important than the specifics of what we do. This photograph by Georgianne Cowan offers a beautiful visual metaphor for being depicted as the kiss of a flowering self. (Courtesy of Georgianne Cowan)

George's parents. As George read through his mother's correspondence, he became irritated. During our session George initially attributed his irritation to his mother's excited but endless "rants" about the trip. As we looked closer, we peeled back a deeper layer. George was irritated at the time frame of his parents' trip, which, he admitted sheepishly, foiled a plan he had been cooking up. George had hoped to "trick" his parents out of feeling upset at the couple's intention not to have Thanksgiving with them but with Sue's parents instead next year. The timing of his parents' trip blocked George's scheme to make an extra, preemptive visit over Easter.

At the time of the email George was feeling pressure from both sides— pressure from his parents to visit often and pressure from his wife to curtail the visits. He had been reflecting on the bubble image between sessions. Perhaps not surprisingly he spontaneously returned to it himself, by describing his current dilemma in bubble terms. "It's like I'm in my own bubble, but everybody else's bubble is crowding in on me, making mine much smaller. Just like with real bubbles, I'm in danger of my bubble merging with the others' if the pressure gets too high" (see Figure 6.9).

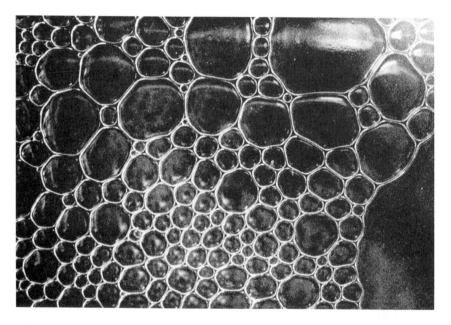

Figure 6.9. This image of foam bubbles beautifully captures the very qualities that George described feeling. There is no possibility for any bubble to exist independently from the others. In fact, each bubble is shaped by completely conforming to the shape of those around it. One gets the feeling of the larger bubbles crowding in on the smaller ones. Meanwhile, everything is smoothed out, because there are no rough edges anywhere. (Courtesy of Richard Taylor)

"Hmmm . . . sounds like a good description of what happened after that last visit to your parents. As I recall, when they got upset at feeling snubbed by your wife, you reflexively defended her, despite actually feeling disturbed by her actions."

"True. I just wanted to make everyone's upset go away. My mother had accused my wife of being the princess who couldn't sleep on the mattress on top of a pea [the couple had experienced the guest bed mattress as too soft, so they had moved it to the floor]. Yet the truth is that both my wife and my mother act like princesses, or maybe I should say they behave like two peas in a pod! My mother is every bit as sensitive to nuance and insult as my wife is. I tried to rationalize Sue's behavior so my mother would feel less hurt and would leave Sue alone."

"You merged bubbles with your mother by ignoring your upset at her for taking offense. And you merged bubbles with Sue by ignoring your upset at your wife for lashing out at your mother."

"Yes, yes, this is all true. So what do I do? As we talk, I can feel myself becoming totally paralyzed. I can't imagine speaking out to anyone about any of this."

"It's hard to know what to do or even what to say if you aren't fully grounded in your own core of how you feel and what you want."

"When everyone else's feelings are this loud, I don't even know *how to know* what I want."

"How about working with those bubbles some more? You could try closing your eyes and picturing yourself in your bubble with everyone else in the family inside their respective bubbles. Let me know what this looks like to you."

Without losing a beat, George closed his eyes and responded almost immediately, "My bubble is pretty small and close to the ground. Sue's is about the same size, and floating right alongside. My mother and father's bubble is much larger, because along with my parents, it contains all my brothers and sisters. Their collective bubble is farther away and much higher up. It seems as if all of the bubbles are filled with hot air, allowing them all to float. But the family bubble keeps rising; it seems in danger of drifting away."

At this point of image articulation, George spontaneously opened his eyes, as if unable to bear the growing distance between bubbles and needing to reconnect with me visually. As before, he looked at me silently, a puzzled look of curiosity pervading his features, as if to wonder what I could see in what he saw. Usually I tend first to explore patients' reactions to products of their own imagination before sharing my own thoughts, images, feelings, or opinions. Yet at that moment, I could not help myself; I felt compelled to blurt out my own reactions (inserting my own bubble filled with hot air!).

"There is something really interesting about your imagery, George! The pattern of tension among the bubbles is opposite to where you started before closing your eyes. Instead of everyone pressing in on your bubble, making yours smaller and more difficult to find your own truths, feelings, and experiences, every bubble here is well separated. And the dangers don't involve merging at all, but quite the opposite. They involved bubbles drifting away from one another. Specifically, your parents and siblings were drifting away from you and Sue. Is it possible that beneath your concerns about upsetting your parents, for fear of *their* anger and rejection, lurks *your* fears of their accepting your wishes, leaving *you* sad at losing the close-knitted bonds of yesteryear?"

"Very possible" was George's response, again bringing that curious mixture of tears and smiles to his face. George's imagery had become a springboard for natural feelings of loss and grief connected with growing up and entering a new phase of life. That George viewed his entire family in a single bubble was a hint that George was less preoccupied with his parents' upset than he realized. This bubble variation revealed George's own distress at individuating into a new marital unit with the power to create a new family tradition. That the bubbles no longer crowded in on one another seemed evidence of increased internal space within George's imagery, cluing him into his own true emotions and desires.

HEALING WITH IMAGINATION

Just as imagination is part of the implicit realm, so, too, is clinical intuition more broadly. George's bubble imagery evolved intuitively from an intersubjective foundation. The imagery emerged as a kind of shared language, forming a collective imaginal space that increased the complexity of our mutual exploration. By adding extra dimensions, imagination is necessary for clinicians to envision a healthier patient, and it is important for patients to open up to novel ways of seeing themselves, others, and the world around them. Pincus and Sheikh (2009) detailed the long history of recruiting imagination in service of emotional and physical healing, dating back to antiquity, whether through shamanic practices, dream interpretation, or Jung's active imagination.

One of Pablo Picasso's most famous phrases was "Every child is an artist. The problem is how to remain an artist once we grow up." Whether or not every child is truly an artist is debatable, yet what is not is that every child is intuitively guided by the internal light of imagination when producing art. All young children are more influenced by inner vision than by outer perception when drawing. This is evident from universal stages of representation (Gardner, 1984), starting with the "tadpole" figure—a circle atop a stick—to indicate the human form. The tadpole figure suggests that what children know on the inside gets completely blended with what they perceive on the outside. As kids mature and progress cognitively, their representation of people tends to look more lifelike. With practice, they can begin to produce true likenesses, including possibilities for three-dimensional renderings.

Interestingly, the tadpole figure is missing in the drawings of autistic art savants such as Nadia, one of the most studied savants due to her unbelievable skill at rendering dynamic, lifelike figures, such as horses and riders. In a recent study (see Figure 6.10), subjects judged her drawings to be more creative than those of Leonardo da Vinci (Ramachandran, 2004). It is likely that, being severely autistic, Nadia lacked a capacity for metaphorical thinking. Ironically this absence of conceptual multisensory blending may have freed up Nadia's perceptual capabilities early for exact representation in a literal way.

Picasso also proclaimed that "everything you can imagine is real." His statement attests to the power of art to materialize in the outer world what begins as inner inspiration. It also holds special relevance and meaning for the endeavor of psychotherapy. On the one hand, many patients present symptoms that can be viewed as a colossal lack of imagination. The hopeless/helpless constellation so typical of depression translates to a failure to envision a future fundamentally different from the past. The frustration associated with feeling stuck or trapped in life translates to the incapacity to imagine a way beyond repetitive patterns. In posttraumatic distress, consistent panic reactions trigger defensive impulses to run, hide, avoid, or disengage through dissociation. Intrusions from past experience block a person's freedom to experience, much less imagine, something different from what life has delivered before.

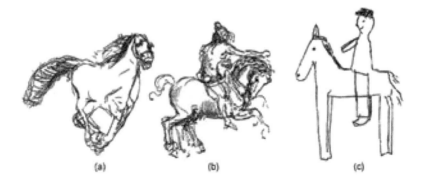

(a)   (b)   (c)

Figure 6.10. (a) Horse drawn by 7-year-old autistic savant Nadia; (b) Horse drawn by Leonardo da Vinci; (c) Horse drawn by a nonautistic 7-year-old child. It is easy to see why viewers preferred the horse drawn by Nadia to that drawn by da Vinci. Nadia's is the most dynamic of all three—in its compacted energy, its quality of movement, and its three-quarter angle to the viewer, giving us the sense the horse could jump out of the page. (Reprinted with permission from Elsevier)

Within psychotherapy, imagination lies at the foundation of healing. This is neither to say that healing is imaginary nor that everything that needs to be healed during psychotherapy is in the mind. Quite the opposite—there is no way to separate the mind from the body, or the body from the brain, including the central and autonomic nervous systems (Marks-Tarlow, 2008a). By the same token, there is no way to separate out the real existence of a patient from the imagination of the therapist. Finally, even at the neurological level, Ramachandran asserted, "This boundary between seeing and imagining has always proved elusive in neurology" (2011, p. 86).

NEURAL FOUNDATIONS FOR IMAGINATION

At its most primitive level, imagination translates to a picture of possible futures. Put this way, imagination is wired into the body of even the most elementary creatures in the form of intention and anticipation. In the premotor cortex of macaque monkeys, canonical cells fire when a monkey either grasps a banana or simply spies one (Iacoboni, 2008). By containing overlapping receptive fields for vision and touch, the monkey's eye becomes effectively linked to its hand through the mapping of a possible future. Because the visual world of an object gets processed in terms of its possibilities for being grasped, the monkey's desires and intentions become built into the very act of perception. Whether or not the monkey actually reaches for the banana matters little, for a potential future automatically gets laid onto what is technically known as a *peripersonal space map*. This is the space that surrounds the body as a map of its potential actions. As inner and outer worlds become inextricably entwined, so, too, do past learning, present circumstances, and potential futures. This nonlinear understanding of time in the body contrasts sharply with the linear timeline to which we have become accustomed.

Much like past and future, perception and action are inseparable in the brain. Also the self and the other are inseparable, partly through the existence of mirror neurons, which also operate in the brain's premotor cortex, among other areas (see Iacoboni, 2008). These neurons fire either when we perform an action or when we see someone else performing that action. Mirror neurons are another "sexy" topic in neurology these days and have been credited with the origins of imitative learning and tool use (Iriki, 2006), communicative gesture, including language (Rizzolatti & Arbib, 1998), and empathic understanding of self and other (Gallese, 2001). Ramachandran (2009) goes so far as to herald mirror neurons as the "greatest discovery in neuroscience since Darwin," attributing to them what is distinct about human culture compared with our closest primate cousins. But keep in mind that mirror neurons do not operate alone, but, with every function listed above, operate in the context of complex neural circuits that implicate a host of brain structures. Although much controversy surrounds the exact functions and significance of canonical and mirror neurons, consider the words of Marco Iacoboni, an early pioneer of mirror neuron research: "Neurons that code for both hand and mouth actions, however, make perfect sense to holistic interpretations of brain functions, in which motor cells are concerned with the *goal* of an action" (2008, p. 15).

Let us consider two aspects of this statement. First, the indivisible operations of perception, action, and interaction indicate a unity in functioning that cannot be parsed reductionistically into separate functions. Second, when the body/mind/brain system is organized in accordance with its potential goals, the organism's past experience becomes inseparable from its present experience as it arcs toward the future, an idea reminiscent of Whitehead's process philosophy (Whitehead, 1929).

This nonreductive, holistic perspective holds as true at the level of single cells firing in the premotor cortex as it does for the entire organism, as well as for the physical and social environments in which organisms operate. Whether we talk about what Iacoboni calls goals, or Walter Freeman (1999, 2000) calls intentionality, imagination in the form of an open future is wired into the basic framework of the brain. The capacity to perceive the present goes hand in hand with a grasp of possible things to come. This form of abstraction coexists with a concrete present, not only in mammals but also in all animal species otherwise lacking in higher cognitive faculties of language, symbol, or formal logic. These proto-forms of imagination are central to perception, implicit learning, and the execution of motor sequences during ordinary brain function even in lower forms of animals.

IMAGINATION INSIDE AND OUTSIDE OF PSYCHOTHERAPY

Within the hierarchy established by evolution, of course, the human imagination reaches the apex. Not only can we envision possible real worlds, but we can also invent impossible unreal ones. From the perspective of clinical intuition, I maintain that imagination represents the highest human faculty through which inner and outer worlds align within a relational context. This loosens up possibilities for change, whether at implicit or explicit levels. During psychotherapy, sometimes imagination precedes reality, as when we can sense the potential of patients to feel better, to change, and to grow, despite horrendous symptoms or how down-and-out they may feel in the moment. This is imagination as an open field of possibilities, eventually to flower however it does. This stands in contrast to the type of imagination where a specific form must be taken. The parallels with parenting are obvious. The use of possible futures helps parents respond to children in attuned fashion so that they may blossom in alignment with their own inner forms versus outer mandates. By contrast, a future too tightly spelled out is the source of much psychopathology, a procrustean bed of demand, where children are straitjacketed into fitting their parents' narcissistic visions for their futures.

Recall the case of Sylvia, introduced in Chapter 4, whose lack of self-agency prevented her from harnessing or even perceiving the incredible potential I immediately intuited from our first moment of contact. I used the synesthetic metaphor of a sputtering jewel to capture Sylvia's capacity to shine and throw off light and positive energy, but only in bits and pieces, before she would get discouraged, lose steam, and collapse in a heap of self-doubt and self-loathing. Sylvia's play with my furniture and her incredible fluency and articulate play with words and concepts immediately revealed to me her enormous creativity.

Over the years as a clinician, I have become convinced that highly creative people must harness their gifts in order to find outer outlets for self-expression or else they will self-destruct, if not die. Sylvia is a case in point. I believe that her degree of self-loathing and her moments of utter despair were directly proportional to collapses in her imaginative sense of her own creative potential. Sylvia easily registered the genius of other people's literary and comedic works. This reflected her "inner" grasp of art directly connected to her own potential for expressive production. But the unrealized gaps between self and other, current self and potential self, were too wide and too painful to bear, especially when Sylvia felt unseen in the eyes of others. Self and other, present and future were not only inextricably bound together, but also inextricably bound up. In intrapsychic space, Sylvia's failure to produce caused her to writhe in the barrenness of creative agony. Within intersubjective space, Sylvia's potential lay curled up like a seed within the relational context of my hope and imaginative capacities to envision a more creative future for her.

IMAGES SPEAK FOR THEMSELVES

As a clinical psychology Ph.D. student at UCLA during the early 1980s, I had the privilege of studying guided imagery with the late Marielle Fuller at the UCLA Neuropsychiatric Institute (currently the Semel Institute). Well into her seventies at the time, if not already in her eighties, Fuller came from France to serve without any advanced degrees as the only "noncredentialed" faculty member within the UCLA Medical School. Fuller became a legend, training hundreds, if not thousands, of psychiatric residents and psychology interns in guided imagery over at least two decades. Fuller had developed a precise sequence of imagery scripts, which she intended to publish but never did before her death a number of years ago. Fuller created and conceived of each image to illuminate a different facet of a person's emotional, relational, and spiritual life. Much as fairy tales crop up independently in different cultures during different eras, Fuller's images have the archetypal feel of being outside of time or authorship.

I would like to share the first image of the meadow: This is a classic to anyone working in the modality of hypnosis or guided imagery. Fuller's method was to describe the full scenario ahead of time, with the patient's eyes open. The script was then self-guided with eyes closed, with Fuller offering a prompt or question at times.

> *When you close your eyes, you find yourself in a meadow, which you are to walk through, describing the meadow in detail. [What does it look like? Smell like? Sound like? What's the temperature, season, and weather? What clothes are you wearing? What kinds of grasses and shrubbery does it contain? Are there trees? Flowers? Any animals?] Somewhere in the field is a shovel. Find it, and once you have the shovel in hand, let it take you to a spot somewhere in the meadow where you are supposed to dig.*
>
> *Keep digging until the shovel hits upon a chest buried somewhere beneath the surface of the ground. Open the chest and take a look at its contents. Take your time going through whatever is inside. When you are finished, if you have taken anything out of the box, return it inside. Put the box back into the hole, and re-bury it using the shovel. Then put the shovel back in its place, walk across the meadow, and exit the place where you entered. When you feel ready, open your eyes and return to the room.*

Fuller met trainees on a weekly basis for 15 weeks, guiding them through a series of images, one at a time. Fuller refrained from discussing the experience afterward, unless someone was deeply upset or needed to talk. Fuller discouraged questions about symbolism or speculations about meaning. Her responses and mandates came out of a strong conviction that the products of imagination work their magic beneath the surface, underneath all words or thoughts, acting on the unconscious to automatically transform our lives, without conscious action, discussion, intervention, or interpretation.

While I sheepishly admit to having little embodied memory for many, if not most, events in my own life, I still remember a good portion of the imagery I produced with Fuller nearly 30 years ago. The experience of working with her has greatly influenced how I use imagery in my own clinical practice, including ways I have been inspired to creatively morph familiar images in unusual ways, such as investigating roots of sexual impotence or innovating custom images of my own for dealing with creative blocks or exam failure. The use of guided imagery is highly intuitive. Even when beginning with a prefabricated image, the journey differs immediately and significantly according to each person's imagination.

When using guided imagery, my own method differs from Fuller's in some respects. Most notably, I do spend time discussing and even interpreting the images and progression of events. However I am careful to separate immersion in the inner journey from any intellectual discussion that follows. I prefer to let a week go by, so that the images have a chance to simmer and incubate in the psyche. This gives people the chance to remain with the subtler emotions and deeper stirrings, as well as to see what dreams might emerge at night. This kind of spacing between immersion and analysis seems to consolidate the experience, including a felt sense of intrinsic meaning and value, into memory.

The image of the meadow provides a topographical metaphor for the psyche that likens qualities of height with conscious accessibility and depth with unconscious, subcortical reaches. Topographical metaphors for the psyche have ancient roots, dating back at least 2,500 years before contemporary psychoanalysis. Consider the words of the ancient Greek philosopher Heraclitis to proclaim the boundlessness of the psyche: "You could not discover the limits of the soul, even if you traveled by every path in order to do so; such is the depth of its meaning."

Likewise, Freud's structural model draws on a topographical metaphor: The superego hovers above head; the conscious ego operates at ground level; and the unconscious id is buried underground. Each of the *depth* psychologies, including Jung's analytical psychology, partakes of a similar metaphor. Consider Jung's famous dream of descending through a house until he reached a hidden chamber in the basement where ancient bones were buried—imagery that inspired Jung's notion of a collective unconscious as distinct from Freud's personal unconscious. I have written previously about central metaphors at the heart of various schools of psychological thought, including those derived from contemporary nonlinear science (see Marks-Tarlow, 2008a).

The image of the meadow follows a long line of predecessors that capitalize on the metaphorical lay of the land to symbolize a vertical relationship between conscious and unconscious processes. The quality of the meadow—how green and fertile it is versus how empty and bleak—represents the patient's immediate state of mind or current quality of life. Access to the shovel and the ease of digging or opening the chest all indicate the nature of people's defenses and resources. The depth and contents of the box, including the experience of understanding and the sense of meaningfulness, symbolize unconscious, implicit levels and their level of integration or disintegration with the conscious self.

Fuller's contention that imagery "speaks for itself" and needs no translation is echoed by others, including James Hillman (1979). One of the reasons that images speak for themselves is because they tend not to lie, while words so easily do. The capacity to lie marks an important developmental step during childhood when children become aware of their freedom to construct imaginary worlds along with their power to fool and deceive adults and other people. When we lie, we consciously spin a yarn we then hand to others. This is possible during guided imagery, because when we do not like the first thing that pops into our heads we can change it deliberately. Yet we can feel the cover-up, just as we can feel the difference between a consciously constructed image and one that emerges unbidden and spontaneously from the unconscious.

Whereas the imagistic right brain has the capacity for error detection and correction, the more verbal left brain does not do so and operates in a vacuum. As McGilchrist (2009) elegantly pointed out, the left brain can only detect errors in internal logic; it therefore depends on the right brain to supply an embodied foundation from which to derive its truths. When the two sides become functionally disconnected from one another, we uncover the full capacity of the left brain to lie.

A wealth of research exists on split-brain patients, beginning from 1960, when the corpus callosum (connecting the two hemispheres) was severed in attempts to stop grand mal epileptic seizures from crossing from one side of the brain to the other (Gazzaniga, 2005). The typical experimental paradigm consists of presenting separate scenarios to the different hemispheres (which also requires splitting each eye's field of vision in half). This results in a left brain that is eager to make conscious, narrative sense by making up reasons for what the right brain indicates in nonconscious, nonverbal ways. As an example, imagine that the right side is shown a picture of a naked woman, which causes the subject to react by blushing. When the left side is asked why his face is red, the person might respond, "Because it's hot in here." Or suppose the right is shown a visual joke leading to laughter. When the left is asked to explain his chuckles, he might respond, "Because you're really funny!"

These occurrences are so frequent, they have led the split-brain researcher Michael Gazzaniga to declare the left hemisphere to be the "interpreter." By this, Gazzaniga meant that the left brain is relentless in making sense out of experience in any way it can, which includes rationalizing and confabulating to cobble meaning out of the emotional side of things. Perhaps Marielle Fuller intuited that words and interpretations of visual imagery can be false compared with the purity of the images themselves. Sadly, perhaps this resistance to words was one reason why Fuller never finished her book. Provocatively, perhaps I am making up Fuller's interior motives even now. If so, then, through writing, I am using the very same facilities to lie that I am trying to expose. Have I just invented another variation of the liar paradox (e.g., this sentence is false: it's true only if it's false and false only if true)? Who knows?

When weaving personal and social narratives, we continually choose the interpretation of events that best suits our perspectives and needs, whether or not it is entirely accurate. Indeed, lots of interesting research suggests that depressed people are more accurate in perceiving conditions in the social world than nondepressed people, even if they are less happy (Lewinsohn, Mischel, Chaplin, & Barton, 1980). One of my dissertation committee members, Shelley Taylor, has researched the value of positive illusions for recovery from life-threatening illnesses (Taylor & Brown, 1994). Ironically, what may start off false can become true in a self-fulfilling way. Depressed people who are more realistic about their chances of surviving cancer might indeed wind up *dead right*. Yet more optimistic people who believe they can beat the odds actually do so more often than hopeless people do. In these cases of mind/body/world unity, the capacity to imagine a healthy future actually helps to usher one in.

IMAGERY AND TRANSFERENCE

I close this chapter with a last iteration of George's bubble imagery, which surrounded yet another email exchange with his mother, this time regarding how to spend his July 4 weekend. Over the previous months, George had made progress with setting limits on the number of trips he and Sue took to visit his parents. Feeling bold, George extended the invitation for his parents to come down to visit them over this holiday weekend instead of vice versa. To George's pleasant surprise, his parents accepted the invitation and even responded graciously to the suggestion of staying overnight in the George and Sue's home.

All seemed to be progressing smoothly until George received a follow-up email. Without George and Sue's knowledge or permission, George's mother had extended an invitation to stay at George and Sue's house to her daughter, George's sister, as well as to her daughter's boyfriend. This crossed a line. George felt his mother had overstepped her rights. He was angry and was determined to respond more directly this time. George wrote an email back, declaring that she had violated his boundaries.

Although George felt satisfied with his bold move, he wound up feeling upset and confused about his mother's subsequent email response, which he brought in to show me. George experienced his mother as having regressed to a third-grade level, using childish language aimed at calming him down. George asked permission to read me the email. The third-grade level of George's request caught my attention, but my intuition told me not to interrupt the flow. I responded, "Sure, go ahead."

"Jeez, George, I am sorry to upset you. Hurray that you also want the whole family to dine at your place. But I do think this boyfriend is here to stay. He and your sister will probably get married and practically already are. If it turns out you are uncomfortable with your sister and her boyfriend staying overnight, they can go to the hotel instead of us. Nothing is set in stone. Please don't stress out. No need for upset."

After hearing what sounded to me like a reasonable discourse, I asked George what he heard in his mother's words. As I suspected, George had read the statement above quite literally, something like, "You better get comfortable with this boyfriend, because he is here to stay. So give him a chance. When your sister and boyfriend arrive at your house, if you feel too uncomfortable for him to stay, we'll change plans on the spot, and he and your sister will go to the hotel instead of us." By contrast, I read the above email as, "No final arrangements have been set; nothing is set in stone. So take the time you need to assess whether or not you are comfortable with your sister's boyfriend. If you decide you are not, then we can prearrange for your sister and her boyfriend to stay in the hotel instead of us."

As soon as I gave George my different sense of his mother's communication, he, too, immediately sensed this as her intended meaning.

"You know, George, when you asked my permission to read your mother's email, I wondered why you had to ask. I had the palpable feeling of a much younger George. Maybe this episode is less about your mother regressing to third grade and more about you doing so. Maybe the act of confronting your mother felt really risky and scary, leaving you feeling like a little kid afraid of retribution. Perhaps this blinded you to the more mature, metaphorical version of what was happening."

"It's funny you should say that. People often do point out how literally I take things."

"That can happen if we live too squarely in the linear, logical side of our brains. But it can also happen when we get stressed out, and our minds go into survival mode and contract from their more expansive, creative aspect."

"I feel bad right now—like I wasted a lot of energy the past two days being upset needlessly. If I hadn't used email, this wouldn't have happened. I would have understood what my mother meant by the tone of her voice as she said it. Then I would have avoided all of this unnecessary confusion and worry."

"You used email because you needed lots of time and space to compose the message. You wanted to write it just as you'd envisioned, without pressure from your mother's immediate presence."

"That's true. If I had called her by phone, I probably wouldn't have confronted her at all. But still, all that space backfired in the end."

"Why do you put yourself down so much right now?"

"I feel like I did after that time I got angry with my parents and confronted them on the phone. I thought I had done a wonderful thing. I came in here expecting a gold star. But you pointed out that I lied to them emotionally, that I had defended behavior in my wife that didn't align with my values."

"So I popped your bubble then, just the way I'm popping it now."

"But you were right then, and you are right now."

"So what? What's so important about being right? Why do you think truth trumps feelings? I may be right in a technical sense, perhaps even in a literal sense, but you are right in an emotional sense. Frankly, especially when it comes to relationships, emotional truths are more basic and important than intellectual ones. If I hurt your feelings and caused you shame, that is a truth we both have to deal with. Frankly, George, in my book (both literally and metaphorically speaking), this is far more important than whether or not I am right in some technical sense."

George both laughed and cried at the same time. Once again, he felt sadness about his own elaborate system of suppressing inner truth, along with happiness and relief in the freedom of self-discovery. But something more had happened through this discussion. We had just broached the transference dimension to George's bubble imagery. Despite my good intentions, he and I had been caught in an enactment. I was much more like his mother than I had realized. Even with every attempt to be sensitive and attuned, I still crowded in on George's bubble, unwittingly helping him to suppress his own perspective and feelings in service of understanding and supporting mine. How ironic that I kept trumping George's perspective. Even in pointing out that his feelings were more important than being right, I still was asserting my perspective over his.

At the end of that session, as we stood up and approached the door, George quipped casually, as if an afterthought, "I really appreciate the images we are using. I think about them often between sessions. It's funny how I often lose the details of exactly what happens during our sessions or what we talk about. But I never forget those images."

WRAP-UP

Clinical intuition not only taps into things as they are—how our patients feel and see the world and how this perspective gets reflected in transference and countertransference dynamics in the room—but it also taps into how things might be—how people might heal and grow and how we might help them do so. Imagination and imagery are primary tools for addressing such potential. Imagination reaches its apex in the human capacity to envision worlds that never were and never will be. Yet a kind of proto-imagination lies curled up implicitly in the very essence of the intentions by which our actions automatically and reflexively arc toward the future.

In this chapter, I have chosen a clinical case that illuminates how imagination can provide clues to more embodied emotional and relational truths than words alone. There is a deeper truth to the free play of imagination that helps to ground us internally so that we may make sound choices and select fitting paths in life.

In order to bring home themes from this chapter, try opening your own imagination in the following ways.

- Find a metaphor that captures your overall feeling about your identity as a therapist. Notice whether the metaphor appeared in words or pictures or some other form.

- Imagine your clinical intuition as an animal. Let that animal lead you to a place of power. When you arrive at your place of power, find a way to communicate with this animal, whether through verbal channels of dialogue or nonverbal channels of mutual gazing, sign language, dance, and so on.
- Pick a difficult case or place where you feel at an impasse with a patient. Seek inner counsel by using guided imagery. Climb a mountain. Find a hut somewhere near or at the top, where you knock on the door to find your guide. Notice what form your inner guide takes, whether it is a wizard, witch, or wizened man. Pose your dilemma and receive a gift from your guide that points toward a solution, with or without words. Do not try to figure anything out. Just let it simmer until later.

The chapter to come expands on the importance of using the inner light of imagination to guide outer paths in life.

CHAPTER 7

Navigating the Seas

A person often meets his destiny on the road he took to avoid it.
                                                                —Jean de La Fontaine

*You have to leave the city of your comfort and go into the wilderness
of your intuition. What you'll discover will be wonderful. What
you'll discover is yourself.*

                                                                —Alan Alda

WHETHER AS AN IMAGE, A FLASH of memory, or a heartfelt song, intuition works hand in hand with imagination by taking the form of embodied metaphor at the heart of self-discovery. Core metaphors begin implicitly with the body's sensory, emotional, and relational experience, helping to provide meaning and direction in life. Early on during infancy, core metaphors related to verticality and balance arise concretely, surrounding the body's physicality; later in life, these metaphors become more symbolic, as cognitive and linguistic capacities are added. Developmentally we *pull ourselves up* in the world, beginning existence from the horizontal position, where we are helpless and dependent on others, to more vertical stances, where we gain balance, agency, and power in the world.

From the start of life, because we are social animals, our explorations of the surrounding environment extend beyond the physical world. We discover our bodies, our selves, and even our surroundings in tandem with exploring the bodies, emotions, and environmental contexts of others.

In this chapter, I address subjectivity as a fully embodied phenomenon, and intersubjectivity as a *spatial and geographical coordinate system that extends through time*. By doing so, I expand on the repertoire of core metaphors from the static postures of balance and verticality (introduced last chapter) in order to include dynamic action and directed movement. Here is my primary stance. Whether in life or in clinical work, to guide ourselves by intuition is to be fully oriented in social space so that we may navigate over time and through experience *from the inside out*, by processing outer information and social cues according to inner vision and dictates. As psychotherapists, the more oriented we are when approaching patients, the more grounded and rooted we stand. This helps us to face difficult emotions and intractable problems, thereby heightening our chances of successful encounters.

I will examine in greater detail how free play helps to integrate the whole of the self, initially by calibrating, that is, aligning and coordinating internal sensory, emotional, behavioral, cognitive, memory, and imaginal faculties. Once these systems are fully calibrated, children are then equipped to navigate their social worlds from the inside out, as illuminated by imagination and guided by intuition. Psychotherapy helps patients restore this early freedom of exploration in order to recalibrate internal systems. This becomes possible when the trusting, secure bond of the therapeutic alliance provides a safe zone in which patients can dream and play in order to find themselves anew.

I begin the chapter with some examples of spatial-temporal metaphors as a prelude to recalling a childhood memory about navigating through physical space. From there, I transition into a clinical story about navigating through social space. I present the case of a young boy whose fantasy play was implicitly designed to illuminate and work through obstacles posed by his parents' conflict-filled marriage. To underscore the importance of free exploration at multiple levels of existence, I turn from there to the value of doodling as an aid to concentration. The stage is fully set for some interpersonal neurobiology. At that point, I will discuss the hippocampus, which internalizes the "what" and "where" and "when" of experience. There is greater value in meandering than in moving in straight, goal-directed lines in order to cultivate a feel for the self in the world from the inside out, through intuition; this is the same for even nonhuman creatures. Yet what initially looks like meandering often reveals purpose-filled patterns from a larger perspective. A final case reveals continuity through the life span, as the unstructured play of childhood flowers into adult self-expression in the workplace.

LOCATING OUR SELVES IN SOCIAL SPACE

During psychotherapy sessions, comments such as these are common:

"I don't understand *where are you going* with that thought?"
"I feel *so lost!*"
"My daughter won't *straighten* herself out."

"I've got to *leave* this marriage, if I'm ever going to *find* myself" (see Figure 7.1).

Each statement contains a metaphor that suggests continuity between the physical spaces occupied by our bodies and the social spaces occupied by our emotional, relational lives. We are so used to discussing our relationships in these concrete terms that we hardly notice the spatial references. How else to describe intimacy but as a feeling of being *close* to someone, perhaps after *breaking down the walls and barriers that separate us*?

From the beginning of life, we occupy an embodied self housed within material space, alongside a social self located in relation to others. The intersubjective field that we cocreate with our parents extends all the way through life, as we continue to rely on others to identify where we stand. Consider this quote from *Eat, Pray, Love* by Elizabeth Gilbert, which of-

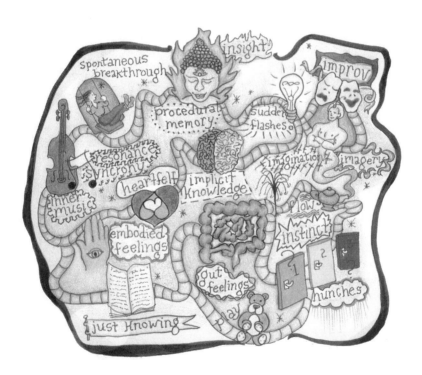

Figure 7.1. Throughout history inner space has been modeled as a territory with spatial extension. Consider Freud's original structural model of the id, ego, and super ego. The unconscious element of the id was buried underground and the conscious ego navigated surface reality, while the lofty ideals and admonitions of the superego's conscience hovered above. To give clinical intuition its own territory helps to make its experience more recognizable and real. (Courtesy of the author)

fers a metaphor of a spacetime grid both for emotions and for empathically *standing in the shoes* of another:

> We were talking the other evening about the phrases one uses when trying to comfort someone who is in distress. I told him that in English we sometimes say, "I've been there." This was unclear to him at first—I've been where? But I explained that deep grief sometimes is almost like a specific location, a coordinate on a map of time. When you are standing in that forest of sorrow, you cannot imagine that you could ever find your way to a better place. But if someone can assure you that they themselves have stood in that same place, and now have moved on, sometimes this will bring hope. (2006, p. 71)

These examples help us to place Lakoff and Johnson's (1980) central metaphors of verticality and balance within a more dynamic context of locomotion and directed action throughout life. By developing an internally grounded sense of direction supplied by inner vision and guidance, we can use intuition to guide the whole of who we are and what we do. This includes how and when to use intuition and how and when to deliberate in a more reasoned and conscious way, including when to consult outside resources. When we move in life from the inside out, guided by the light of intuition, we position the holistic, integrating faculties of the right brain to organize the piecemeal, fragmented style of the left brain. This allows us to chart the course of our lives in such a way that intuition remains the master, while deliberation functions both as its servant and as its gift.

DRIVING MYSELF INTO CONFUSION

As I began writing this chapter, a childhood scene kept popping into my head. I was tempted to brush it away until I realized its relevance. Once again, my unconscious instincts proved cleverer than any conscious intentions. What follows may be my earliest coherent memory. I was driving through the countryside with my mother. These were the days before car seats, so I was permitted to sit in the front seat. Normally I loved to look out the window and watch the scenery rushing by. On this particular day I turned to watch my mother instead and became riveted by the motion of her hands and arms. I could see all the tiny tweaks, twists, and turns of how she was steering the wheel, first clockwise, then counterclockwise. Some movements were smooth and long, and others jerky and short. Always her hands changed direction, as the steering wheel jumped about, ever in motion.

I looked and looked, trying to discern a pattern within it all. As hard as I tried, I simply could not find a consistent trend from one minute to the next. At first I was entranced by the erratic cadence. Then I started to *think about* what was happening just a little too hard (a recurrent problem). I began to imagine myself as my mother sitting behind that very same wheel. And this was all it took for me to fly into a panic.

"Uh oh!" I thought. "If I tried to drive, surely we would crash. I wouldn't be able to do it! Without a clear pattern to all those little movements, how could I remember the sequence by heart? If every journey is as complicated as this one, my mother must be a genius, and I will *never* learn to drive!" What started in joy and wonderment rapidly deteriorated into helpless despair.

As I look back, the train of my young mind presaged my continuing confusion over left-brain, consciously directed functioning versus the right-brain, implicitly organized response. Perhaps this confusion stemmed from being a left-handed creature in a right-handed world, where my hands continually competed with each other for the right to use the scissors or a hammer, to play ping-pong, or to sew with a thread and needle. Or perhaps my panic stemmed from feeling rather alone and insecure in the world from the start, even in the presence of my parents. Whatever its source, the error in thinking produced by an immature mind is obvious to me now (see Figure 7.2). Those tweaks and twists were not some elaborate sequence that needed conscious learning, memorization, and performance. Rather they emerged out of a broad base of implicit learning that granted my mother an intuitive feel for how to drive, combined with minute-to-minute attention to details and incorporation of feedback, which permitted accuracy in my mother's perception and sound judgment in our directed motion.

From a very young age I struggled to understand how people made their way through the world. Sadly, I began life feeling woefully ill-equipped in this department. Happily, dogged persistence on my part has led to some hard-earned feelings of mastery and security. The next clinical tale presents a little boy whose early play appears designed to counteract just this sort of panic and self-doubt.

ALL HAIL THE MILK KING

Carl was so delayed in his speech that when his words were still sputtering out one by one well into his third year, his mother became worried. She sent her son to speech therapy, amidst some scary prognoses. But the uneven pace by which all children develop brings danger in comparing one child with another too closely, even when using age-graded norms. Development in children is universally highly idiosyncratic, and what starts out slow will often shoot ahead. This is exactly what happened with Carl. When his words did start to flow, they poured forth in a gush to saturate the rich field of the young boy's imagination.

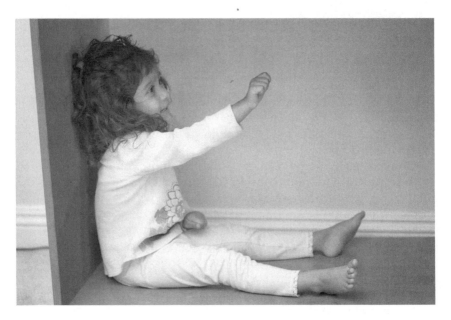

Figure 7.2. This little girl has turned the nook under her mommy's desk into a fantasy zone for driving an imaginary car. Notice how comfortable and relaxed she is. We can almost see a fantasy destination in her eyes. What a contrast with my own early panic at the thought of driving! (Courtesy of Remy Ashe)

As a first grader, Carl loved war games. His fantasy play often included huge armies operating within elaborate chains of command. Carl frequently drew his father into his games. Carl's father, who also had a rich imagination, took great pride and delight in nurturing his son's creativity. One common variation of the war game used empty drink bottles and consisted of the Milk Army pitted against the Soda Army. One day, as they played together, Carl's father started to move some of his soldiers forward aggressively. Carl abruptly stopped him with a question.

"What are you doing, Dad?"

"I'm coming in for the attack."

"No," said Carl, "that's not what's supposed to happen. The two armies aren't supposed to fight!"

"They aren't supposed to fight? Well, then what *is* supposed to happen?" asked Carl's father, flashing his son a puzzled but interested look.

"The General of the Milks wants to visit the General of the Sodas."

"Really? Why does he want to do that?"

"He's going to bring gifts and samples of milk with him," replied Carl in a matter-of-fact tone.

"What's his mission?" asked Carl's father.

"He's trying to make peace. Dad, you've got to understand something. The idea isn't to 'win' the war. Everybody loses if there's a real war. The idea is to 'win the soda general over' to the benefits of drinking milk. That way, maybe he will stop slugging down all that unhealthy soda."

This story was reported to me in a doting anecdote by Carl's father, my patient in psychotherapy. A little background is in order. Dad was a bit of a "health fanatic," a vegetarian for years who was thin and trim. Dad was acutely aware of every vitamin and morsel he put into his body and he prided himself greatly on healthy eating. Carl's mom, on the other hand, focused concerns in other areas, including work. Mom fretted easily and worried ceaselessly, especially when changes were afoot or the future felt uncertain.

At the time of this story, Dad was slated to be laid off, which worried and angered Carl's mom. Huge gaps in her own father's employment history haunted her, triggering fears of financial ruin, despite ample reserves in the bank, a good severance package in the works, and few gaps in her husband's financial contributions to date. Whereas Carl's dad was upbeat and optimistic, Carl's mom was prone to worry and catastrophic thinking. Consciously she wished to protect the family by foreseeing problems and focusing on whatever could go wrong. Unfortunately, the strategy easily backfired, causing problems instead.

Carl's mother had taken to snacking ceaselessly as a way to deal with her worries. She was steadily gaining weight, eating at fast food restaurants for convenience, and indulging in junk food for comfort. To top it off, Carl's mother was too moody and restless to join the rest of her family for sit-down dinners. This only contributed to her husband's extreme upset at not feeling more fully supported by his wife, especially during a time of transition. Secretly Carl's father fantasized about leaving the marriage. Yet his love for Carl inevitably pulled him back into the fray.

Carl admired his dad greatly and followed in his footsteps in many ways. Carl loved to read the ingredients on jars, boxes, and foods purchased at the store, and he soon understood the difference between saturated and unsaturated fats. Likewise, he carefully considered what he put into his young body. Carl's interests in nutrition, reinforced by his elementary school education and his adoration for his dad along with concern for his mother, were all evident in his imaginary play. Carl's clever peace-making war game represented not only the intractable problems he perceived between his parents, but it was also a clever way to solve them based on empathy and communication, which were two ingredients sorely lacking in the household.

The holistic brilliance of Carl's play reflected intuition operating at its highest level. In the silent war between his parents, Carl absorbed the intensity of his parents' conflict. He clearly accepted the hidden mandate to adopt the role of go-between and ambassador. Carl displayed an implicit understanding of where each parent stood, indicating his disapproval for the kinds of high stakes typical in a win/lose paradigm. During marital conflict, one person winning at the expense of the other surely leads to the whole family losing. Out of exquisite empathy for his dad, plus a desire to "win over" his mother to greater health, intimacy, play, and communication, Carl devised a clever plan to conduct the war by avoiding fighting altogether. Instead, he became solution-focused via communication and compromise. By directing his own hope and optimism in this manner during play, Carl displayed powerful leadership skills within his family system.

Inside Carl's play space, we detect the *transitional space* identified by Winnicott (1971) that exists *between fantasy and reality*. Carl's game contained realistic bits of his parents' struggle, imaginatively pointing toward a new future, seen (or scene) through the lens of Carl's subjectivity. By representing serious, real-world concerns on the safe turf of play, Carl used the play of intuition to feel his way through his parents' struggles, offering solutions on his own terms. By drawing his father regularly into the game, Carl continually re-charmed his dad with his clever fantasy life, implicitly reinforcing his father's urges to stay in the marriage. By occasionally drawing his mother into the game, Carl helped to lighten up her mood while bringing her into the very same arena where dad was so comfortable.

Had Carl been more traumatized by the conflict between his parents, his free play likely would have been less complex and coherent. Fortunately, the boy was securely attached to each parent as an individual. This provided a safe platform to navigate his parents' potentially explosive differences.

OODLES OF DOODLES

Carl's story helps us understand the value of attacking issues from the side sometimes. Intuitively directed free play often addresses serious business at implicit levels, while providing the leading edge of development where serious cognitive, social, emotional, and behavioral skills can be learned. Child therapists understand this implicitly when they witness and encourage their youngest patients to return to traumatic situations through the use of puppets or stuffed animals.

When intuitive faculties of the right brain take the lead, precisely because they are holistic and nonlinear in nature, issues are approached sideways, sometimes in very meandering ways. This sideways approach differs greatly from the direct, straightforward, and linear style of the left brain. But precisely because the right brain is specialized to process and absorb new things, it behooves us to have patience and respect its meandering, circuitous style. Here is an example to bring home this point.

On March 12, 2009, National Public Radio ran a story about Tony Blair, the British prime minister at the time, who had appeared on a panel at the World Economic Forum in Davos along with Bill Gates, Bill Clinton, and the rock star Bono. When the event was over, a journalist wandered onto the stage where he discovered papers left behind, near Blair's seat. The papers contained circles, triangles, boxes, and arrows—in short, they were covered in doodles. The journalist brought his treasures to a British graphologist who concluded the prime minister was "struggling to maintain control in a confusing world," was "not rooted," and even worse, was "not a natural leader, but more of a spiritual person, like a vicar." The story spread like wildfire through the British newspapers. Two days later, No. 10 Downing Street weighed in with an important announcement: It was not Tony Blair who created those doodles. Rather, it was Bill Gates.

As a doodler, Gates is in good company, alongside Lyndon Johnson, Ralph Waldo Emerson, Ronald Reagan, and Barack Obama. Who among us has not doodled at some point in our lives? The NPR story next turned to analysis of the impulse to doodle by consulting Jackie Andrade, a psychology professor at the University of Plymouth. Andrade explained that when people are bored, their brains remain very active and use up lots of energy. Put more technically, this continual activity of areas of the brain, especially the dorsolateral and medial prefrontal cortex, is known as the *default mode*.

Because the brain is designed to constantly process information, non-stimulating environments pose a problem: "You wouldn't want the brain to just switch off, because a bear might walk up behind you and attack you; you need to be on the lookout for something happening." A brain that lacks sufficient stimulation scavenges for something to occupy its attention. One common solution is to manufacture its own material by turning to daydreams and fantasies. But these also take an enormous amount of energy, as well as competing for cognitive attention. Doodling is a far better choice. Doodling provides just enough cognitive stimulation to prevent the mind from totally tuning out and retreating into fantasy.

Andrade (2009) tested her theory by playing a long, boring tape of a telephone message to subjects. Half were given a doodling task, and half were not. When the tape ended, subjects were tested on retention. Doodlers remembered 29% more information than nondoodlers did. The NPR story concluded that "doodling . . . is a very good strategy for the next time you find yourself stuck on a slow-moving panel with an aging rock star and verbose former president" (see Figure 7.3).

SEEING THROUGH MOVING

While Bill Gates may have dropped out of Harvard in order to pursue other interests, clearly he is no slacker. It may be surprising to learn that far from indicating a wandering mind, doodling oftentimes aids in concentration. This is one variation of the broader theme of this book that play is a vital ingredient for serious business. Meanwhile there is a

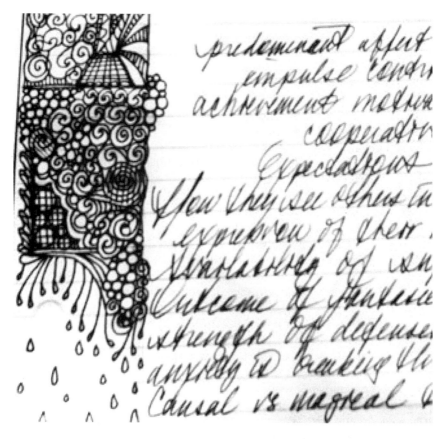

Figure 7.3. Here is the doodle of a graduate student who sat in one of my neurobiology classes. Since the birth of her three children and all that life has entailed since, my student has struggled to focus attention. During my class, her pen moved continually, doodling to enhance attention in a hopefully not too boring class. (Courtesy of the doodler)

subtheme here that things are often not as straightforward as our logical minds might dictate or wish. Many more surprises such as these lie ahead as nonlinear science continues to infuse our perspective (see Marks-Tarlow, 2008a).

There is a classic but incorrect view of the young child's receptive mind that dates all the way back to ancient Greece, setting forth the notion of the *tabula rasa*, or blank slate. This underlying metaphor suggests that input from the environment gets imprinted onto a child's initially empty mind through sensory data that are passively taken in from the eyes, ears, touch, and other senses. If the mind is a blank slate, and we fill this slate with squiggles and doodles, this should leave little room for other, more important information. But as indicated, the metaphor leads us down a false alley (I could not resist introducing that spatial twist). Not only does the existence of a default mode suggest the mind is not passive, but rather is active all the time, but also, the body plays a starring role in how the body/mind/brain system creates information.

There is nothing inherently meaningful about sensory data. Instead the capacity to derive meaning from the senses is experience-dependent through interaction with the world. In many cases, the capacity to derive meaningful perception emerges during critical developmental windows, when the senses get calibrated (or lined up and coordinated) in accordance with feedback supplied by the body as it moves physically through the world. Take vision as an example. In a classic study by Held and Hein (1963), two newborn kittens were yoked together in a carousel that circled round and round in a visually restricted environment. One kitten had free locomotion, while the other was passively carried in a basket. They shared similar views of the outside environment, yet only the kitten with free locomotion developed normal vision (see Figure 7.4).

These same conditions hold for people. This explains why restoring vision to a congenitally blind adult can be futile (Ostrovsky, Andalman, & Sinha 2006). Despite normal sensory signals, the critical window for internal alignment of faculties, or calibration, has passed. Left in the "blooming, buzzing confusion" William James mistakenly attributed to newborn babies, many of these individuals choose to return to blindness.

Whether in kittens or people, movement-produced sensory feedback during early critical periods is necessary to enable visually guided behavior. Put slightly differently, in order to navigate the world according to outside-in cues delivered through sight alone, our bodies must first have ample opportunities to feel their way through the visual environment from the inside out. Furthermore, these same conditions that hold true for vision also apply more broadly to how we become oriented culturally and socially within intersubjective space.

NAVIGATING OUTER WORLDS

The hippocampus is a bilateral (two-sided, one in each cerebral hemisphere) brain structure located deep within the medial temporal lobe, near the amygdala (see Figures 7.5 and 7.6). Both the hippocampus and amygdala are important for encoding human memory. Whereas the amygdala lays down implicit, nonconsciously processed emotional memories, the hippocampus helps us to navigate in space by identifying where we are and what is going on, as well as to lay down the explicit, consciously processed tracks of autobiographical memory. The architecture of the human hippocampus is a bit like a random graph (Buzsáki, 2006), specializing in what is unique and arbitrary to facilitate the idiosyncratic storehouse of

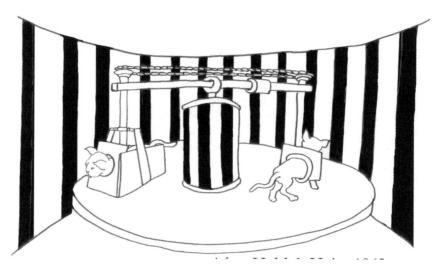

Figure 7.4. This is a rendering of the yoked kitten experimental paradigm, published by Held and Hein in 1963. In this study, two kittens experience the same visual environment, yet only the one that is free to move through the environment developed normal vision. This classic study was proof that perception is not the passive reception of visual stimuli. Instead, perception requires the sensorimotor feedback from full body immersion. (Courtesy of the author)

memories possessed by each one of us. This meandering structure, containing both limbic and nonlimbic aspects, contrasts sharply with sensory areas of the cerebral cortex, which are more hierarchically ordered. By being stacked into neat columns and layers, the sensory areas are best able to extract invariant, stable order from the outside environment.

György Buzsáki is a neuroresearcher especially interested in the rat's hippocampus. Buzsáki's lab has spent decades studying neuronal firings of individual place cells in the hippocampus. In rats, this area of the brain is essential to becoming oriented in the environment in order to navigate successfully through physical space. Buzsáki (2006) identified two distinct phases by which rats become oriented. During the first stage, as *rats freely explore* the environment, individual place cells in the hippocampus fire in recognition. This creates an ongoing, one-dimensional stream of present-centered experience that Buzsáki likens to the nautical technique of *dead reckoning*. Just as early sailors kept track of their direction, speed, and time of travel on an ongoing basis, rats begin by feeling their way through the environment. By recursively enfolding interoceptive feedback (internal organs), along with exteroceptive feedback (smell, taste, touch, sight, sound, balance) as well as proprioceptive feedback

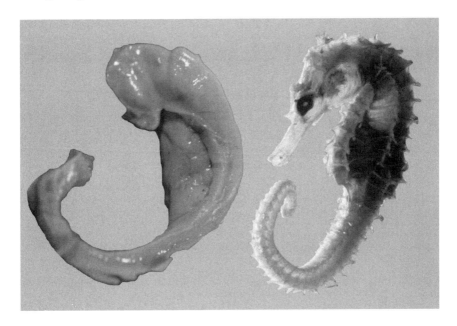

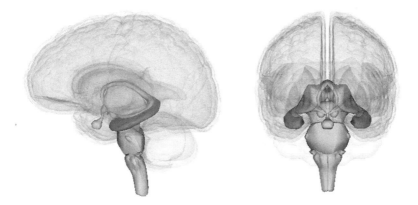

Figure 7.5. Top: Preparation of a human hippocampus alongside a sea horse. The word "hippocampus" derives from Latin; hippo means "horse," kampos means "sea" (Public domain, courtesy of Laszlo Seress). Bottom: Hippocampus, side and front view. Although the hippocampus lies beneath the cortex, it can be considered a cortical infolding that is more ancient and primitive in structure. The hippocampus contains only three layers compared with the six layers that form the neocortex. (From Anatomography, website maintained by Life Science Databases [LSDB]).

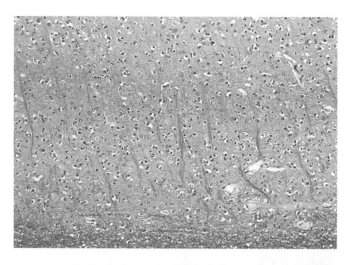

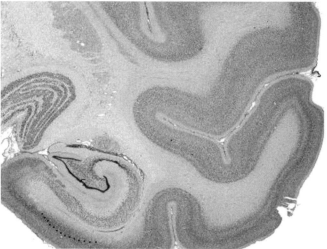

Figure 7.6. Top: Reveals the regular, hierarchical cell structure of the visual, sensory cortex, which can be divided into neat vertical columns and horizontal layers. Bottom: Reveals the swirling, irregular cell structure of the hippocampus, designed to record personalized experience. Whereas the sensory cortex stabilizes perception of the outside environment by extracting invariant features, the hippocampus is laid out more like the RAM (random access memory) of a computer to facilitate unlikely interconnections and highlight idiosyncratic elements of experience. (Public domain, courtesy of brainmaps.org)

(whether the body is moving, where various body parts are relative to one another), internal systems aligned and integrated (i.e., calibrated) at the same time that external maps are created of the outside world.

Once calibration is achieved in this manner, rats then have a reliable foundation for switching modes. During the second phase of orientation that Buzsáki called *map-based navigation*, rats then can travel through the environment *according to external landmarks and recognizable cues* such as the sight of a water dish or a familiar running wheel. Again drawing on a nautical metaphor, Buzsáki likened this stage to sailors' *landmark navigation*. When mathematics advanced to the point where complicated calculations could be made of a ship's whereabouts relative to the positions of celestial features like the stars, sun, and moon, there was no longer an ongoing need to continually track position. This freed sailors to update their whereabouts infrequently, only once or twice a day.

Buzsáki's research led to an important conclusion. Rats need freedom to explore the environment from the inside out, through touch aligned with other sensorimotor faculties, before they can orient and navigate from the outside in, according to external visual cues alone. But there is an additional nonlinear twist to this rat tale/tail. When these rodents were restricted to running along tracks in straight lines while exploring, they failed to orient fully to their environments. Because place cells in the hippocampus are omnidirectional, they need to be triggered from multiple angles in order to establish a two-dimensional grid of external space. Only by enjoying the full freedom *to meander chaotically and approach any point from any other point in space* can rats truly internalize the "what" and "where" of outer experience. But so far, in these rats at least, the "when" has been left out of the picture.

NAVIGATING DOWN MEMORY LANE

In a previous paper (Marks-Tarlow, 2011) I suggested that people go through these same two phases of orienting and navigating in social space that rats go through in physical space. In other words, people first must calibrate internal sensory, motor, affective, cognitive, behavioral, and imaginal systems through dead reckoning (orienting from the inside out by internal touch and feel) in order to later switch to map-based navigation (traveling from the outside in according to external cues), using the hippocampus all the while.

Does the human hippocampus work like this? Researchers have determined that the human hippocampus helps us to navigate through ongoing experience by laying down personal memory tracks partly because damage to this brain structure results in profound memory problems. Perhaps the most famous case involved a man named Henry Gustav

Molaison, known as HM for short. Following severe epilepsy that likely stemmed from a bicycle accident at age 9, in 1957 at age 19 HM had most of his temporal lobe bilaterally removed. From that point until his death in 2008, HM was visited by a steady stream of neurologists fascinated by the workings of his brain and mind.

Because HM's implicit memory was completely intact, he could play bingo, do crossword puzzles, and enjoy socializing with his caretakers. In other words, HM's body could remember complicated behavioral and social sequences that were learned before and even after his surgery (Newhouse, 2008). Yet because of the loss of his hippocampus, HM was unable to convert short-term events into new long-term memory. He could not remember what he ate for breakfast that day, could not state the current day of the week or year, and he could not cite the names of caretakers who had been his daily companions for the years after his accident.

How does the human line of research on autobiographical memory in the hippocampus converge with the line of research on rats' place cells in the same brain structure? The missing link is the temporal dimension or the "when" of experience, which Buzsáki figured out. By tracking the firing of an individual place in the rat hippocampus, Buzsáki's lab attended to time at an implicit level, through noting precisely "when" these cells would fire as the rat reached a particular location in space. This contrasts with autobiographical memory in people, where the dimension of time becomes more explicit. In other words, rats using the "when" of neural firing to track how their bodies move through physical space (the "what" and "where") transitioned through evolution into people tracking how their minds move through social space and time (the "what," "where," and "when"). By attending to simultaneity (see Vogel, Rössler, & Marks-Tarlow, 2008) in neural firing in the temporal dimension, Buzsáki directly linked research on rats navigating physical space with research on humans navigating social space (that is, personal memory).

What was implicit within mammalian hippocampal navigation, or the linking of time with place, became explicit within human hippocampal memory. Recent research (Yin & Troger, 2011) indicates that the hippocampus plays an important role in keeping accurate and reliable timing within the brain broadly. This is an excellent example of how an evolutionarily earlier brain structure became co-opted for a different use, including new, emergent function in the form of human episodic memory.

I believe that therapists must consider this research for two reasons. First, the findings help provide continuity between the concrete nature of physical space with the symbolic nature of social space. Fluid boundaries between physical and social dimensions of life are evident for any therapist who addresses mind/body issues. For example, there is great power in interpreting the symbolic significance of physical symptoms (a top-down approach), while there is also great power in finding that the body correlates to emotional issues (a bottom-up approach). Second, Buzsáki's findings restore the body to the center of memory, not to mention clinical work, even for talk therapists. As noted previously, there is a growing trend among therapists, especially those interested in trauma, to pay attention to how the body holds symptoms, emotions, and healing as well. The body, especially its autonomic and limbic functioning, is likewise at the center of clinical intuition. It is through the body's feel of our social world that we learn to remain oriented within each clinical moment. This helps us to harness implicit faculties necessary to navigate through the next moment, however uncertain we may feel.

When therapists are fully oriented in social space (one outcome of secure or earned attachment), then we are more open to exploring unchartered territory with patients. We are more willing to take emotional risks in the face of potentially dangerous, but possibly enriching, situations. This can help us to face emotionally challenging dilemmas with patients, where intense levels of fear or anger might otherwise be disruptive. Because we are aligned and grounded internally, we are more receptive to incoming information. We can make better sense of multiple sensory streams, even at high levels of arousal, while incorporating and responding to continual feedback. All of this helps us to move through novel encounters more spontaneously, fluidly, and gracefully. This enhances internal grounding and self-trust on which our social sensitivity and sound judgment depend.

RHYTHMS IN THE BRAIN

At a physiological level, in order to make the leap between single place cell firings within the rat hippocampus to whole-structure operation within the human hippocampus, brain rhythms become important order parameters (organizing variables) for large-scale neuronal behavior. In the mammalian brain, a spectrum of different waves coexist, each operating at a different frequency (see Figure 7.7). Taken together, these rhythms simultaneously generate electrical impulses that help to link emotional, cognitive, attentional, imaginal, and behavioral processes.

Here is a rough guideline of rhythms for the human brain, from slowest to fastest:

1. Delta (1 to 3 cycles per second) is an inhibitory wave, particularly active during sleep, that helps to synchronize and fine-tune other rhythms.
2. Theta (4 to 7 cycles per second) assists us in conscious orientation, governing how we allocate attention outward, into the world around us, as well as how we allocate attention inward, as when we daydream.
3. Alpha (8 to 11 cycles per second) involves rest and relaxation as we turn inward.

Brain Frequencies

DELTA   = 1 - 3   Hertz
THETA   = 4 - 7   Hertz
ALPHA   = 8 - 11 Hertz
BETA   = 12 - 29 Hertz
GAMMA   = 30 - 50 Hertz

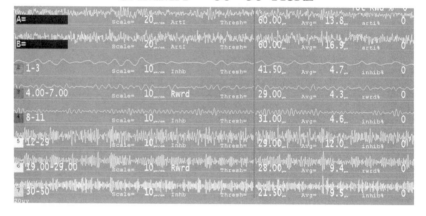

Figure 7.7. These brain-wave frequency bands utilizing an EEG neurofeedback system were taken from a nontraining evaluation. (Courtesy of Jaclyn M. Gisburne, Ph.D.)

4. Beta (12 to 29 cycles per second) comes online when the brain is actively aroused and engaged in mental activities.
5. Gamma (30 to 50 cycles per second) binds different parts and areas of the brain during real-time events, providing coordination dynamics between synchronous and asynchronous events.

Hippocampal theta was the first cortical rhythm observed in the mammalian brain and was discovered within immobile, anesthetized rabbits. Grastyán (Grastyán, Lissák, Madarász, & Donhogger, 1959) later demonstrated the significance of the theta rhythm for the orienting reflex within moving cats. As more research was conducted on the theta brain wave, the list of behavioral correlates grew longer, eventually including the whole of motor output. This led Vanderwolf (1969) to set forth the voluntary movement hypothesis of theta, whereas Grastyán speculated that theta is an invariant correlate of play. Grastyán's conclusion brings us full circle, back to the importance of play. If the theta rhythm is critical for orienting, for allocating conscious attention, for voluntary responding, as well as for play, then theta appears to signal transition and coordination zones between inner and outer landscapes. Indeed, evidence accumulates from other sources that navigation, memory, and the capacity to envision the future plus landscapes of imagination all implicate the same underlying neurobiology (Knox, 2010).

NAVIGATING FROM THE INSIDE OUT
THROUGH FREE PLAY

When it comes to early development, there are a number of ways by which the fetus, child, and adult become oriented within their bodies and within the outside environment: through the inner equilibrium of our ears; through the touch of our bodies; and through the expression and reception of emotions and through the gaze of our eyes among other senses. Those immersed in yoga or in various martial arts would likely add connection with our core as a fourth source of balance and orientation.

What we do concretely with our bodies, we also do symbolically in social space by finding our place among others, as if locating our position as a geographic node. Consider another quote from Elizabeth Gilbert's first memoir, inspired by the Indonesian portion of her trip:

> The whole idea of Bali is a matrix, a massive and invisible grid of spirits, guides, paths and customs. Every Balinese knows exactly where he or she belongs, oriented within this great, intangible map. Just look at the four names of almost every Balinese citizen—First, Second, Third, Fourth—reminding them all of when they were born in the family, and where they belong. You couldn't have a clearer social mapping system if you called your kids North, South, East and West. Mario, my new Italian-Indonesian friend, told me he is only happy when he can maintain himself—mentally and spiritually—at the intersection between a vertical line and horizontal one, in a state of perfect balance. For this, he needs to know exactly where he is located at every moment, both in his relationship to the divine and to his family here on earth. If he loses that balance, he loses his power. (2006, p. 227)

As an aside, my husband and I honeymooned on Bali and were so enchanted by this system that our first child's middle name is Wyan, derived from the Balinese name for a first-born boy. This Balinese social mapping system situates the individual self in relationship to God and family as it relates to a person's earthly presence.

From a neurobiological standpoint, the self is embodied, meaning that it is encased in a body that is concretely embedded in a physical, social, and cultural environment. Meanwhile, as discussed previously, the self is emotionally based (see Damasio, 1999; Varela, Thompson, & Rosch, 1991). The "primary affective core" (Emde, 1983) involves nonconscious, preverbal, and implicit processes that are present in the womb (Schore, 1994;

Siegel, 1999). This affective core is fed and developed through a steady stream of present-centered sensory, affective, interoceptive (sensing the internal world), and exteroceptive (sensing the external world) experiences that are derived from interaction with the physical and social world. These experiences are composed of basic feelings of *aliveness* (Fogel & Garvey, 2007) and *embodied self-awareness* (see Fogel, 2009). Another parallel stream central to the self involves *conceptual self-awareness,* which develops later, beginning in the second year of life. This more conscious, language- and reason-based aspect consists of labels, judgments, narratives, autobiographical memories, intellectual descriptions, and defenses. Each stream of self-awareness implicates distinct brain structures, circuits, time scales, and neurophysiological underpinnings. Ideally the two function in an integrated manner. As proposed next, play may help to align these separate streams.

Whereas rats need the freedom to explore any point in space from any other point to become oriented from the inside out, so, too, do children need the freedom to explore any point in social space from any other point through unstructured play in order to become oriented from the inside out (Marks-Tarlow, 2010). This is one reason why children return to the same game over and over, introducing minor and sometimes major variations in the rules, roles, and relationships. As I have written previously,

> twists and turns in play narratives not infrequently trigger a 180-degree turn into self-contradiction. One minute a child, as fireman, urgently rushes to the scene of a blazing fire intent on saving a house from the flames. The next minute, our little hero morphs into a villain determined to toss the house into the fire instead. The co-existence of such opposites fires up children's passions within a safe environment, where nothing really burns, and everything fuels flames of creative inspiration. (2010, p. 41)

As another example, one day Sarah is the doctor who heals Billie as a patient; the next day Billie is the doctor, but patient Sarah dies; on the third day Billie is an ambulance driver, while Sarah is a mortician. Only by examining each role from the perspective of every other can children fully understand and internalize the medical system as a whole. This key developmental finding of the researcher Brian Sutton-Smith (1979, 1997) also relates to the concept of social orientation. By exploring each point in social space from the perspective of many other points, all sensory, emotional, behavioral, cognitive, and imaginal systems become aligned and calibrated. Once these systems are fully oriented, children can switch to Buzsáki's second phase of landmark navigation, by which external information and social cues are processed according to inner dictates and intuition.

Through free play, children not only gain social skills of coordinating language, action, and imagination in a social setting, but they also learn how to relax and become fully oriented in the present moment using full engagement of all faculties (see Figure 7.8). This "inside out" navigation sets the stage for later periods of "outside in" development when children fall in love with facts about the world.

In the same paper (Marks-Tarlow, 2010), I further proposed that this two-step transition from inside-out to outside-in navigation amounts to an alignment between Fogel's (2009) parallel streams of self-awareness—the earlier embodied flow of right-hemisphere, implicit processes and the later developing conceptual flow of left-brain, explicit processes. As the two streams become aligned through the resonance of entrained timing as well as through feedback carried across the corpus callosum, a minute-to-minute subcortical stream of body-based information can feed into and ground the more disembodied, conceptual flow of words, thoughts, and evaluations.

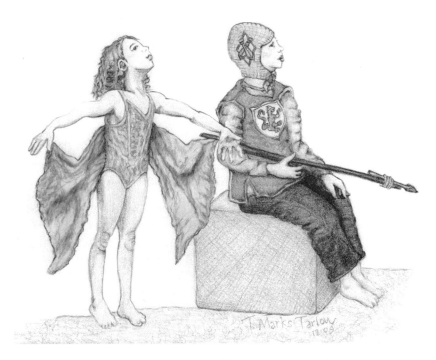

Figure 7.8. When children are guided by the free play of imagination, they proactively explore their social worlds, guided by intuition and motivated by curiosity, joy, and passion. Inner faculties and outer worlds align. Agency and identity are discovered. During psychotherapy, even as adults the free play of imagination helps to provide a safe context for introducing novelty and realigning emotional, motivational, cognitive, and behavioral faculties. (Courtesy of the author)

Only if these two streams of self-awareness are fully aligned can imagination serve as an inner beacon for outer travels throughout life. In less successful cases where inner calibration is not achieved, the two streams of embodied and conceptual self-awareness do not line up, which might lead either to somatic or social disorientation, perhaps providing a context for yet another Gilbert spatial metaphor for emotional processes:

> When you're lost in those woods, it sometimes takes you a while to realize that you *are* lost. For the longest time, you can convince yourself that you've just wandered a few feet off the path, that you'll find your way back to the trailhead any moment now. Then night falls again and again, and you still have no idea where you are, and it's time to admit that you have bewildered yourself so far off the path that you don't even know from which direction the sun rises anymore. (2006, p. 48)

Rather than serving as a beacon into a real future, when our inner faculties are not aligned and integrated, imagination can fail to serve us, or it can function defensively instead by walling off and protecting a fragile self, resulting in a constricted, suppressed, repressed, or dissociated affective core (see Figure 7.9; Fogel, 2009). Remember the case of Suzette from Chapter 2 who came to California to become an actress, but then wound up arrested for prostitution? Suzette had wandered so far off the path that the only acting she did was pretending everything was okay when it really was not.

NAVIGATING FROM THE INSIDE OUT
DURING PSYCHOTHERAPY

What I have just described is how intuitive faculties get established during childhood play. I suggested that the safety of play combined with the freedom to let our imaginations fly enables children to align and coordinate their inner worlds with their outer worlds. Once inner faculties are calibrated in this way, children can process new information that comes from external sources while navigating novel social situations in alignment with internal guidance.

These very same principles hold for the operation of clinical intuition. As therapists, we need the freedom to navigate clinically from all angles. One thing this implies is the importance of approaching the profession from a position of having played both roles—that of patient as well as that of therapist. Here, playing the role of patient is not solely in service of healing psychopathology or even getting hold of countertransference vulnerabilities, but as much to provide a holistic view of the system, which lends greater fluidity in understanding the various parts.

There is another important conclusion to draw from this perspective. The deepest levels of change are possible only when therapists and patients have the freedom to meander through the intersubjective field

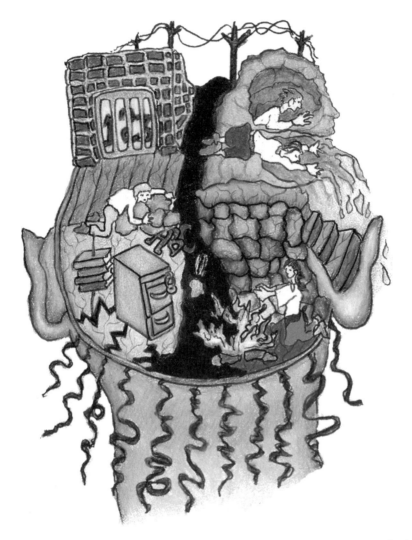

Figure 7.9. This drawing of the brain's two hemispheres as physical locations was requested by the mother of an adopted, 8-year-old Ukrainian child. The child suffered from radical attachment disorder. The drawing's gaps, floods, walls, and downed telephone lines became a means for him to understand what was happening in his brain during highly dysregulated periods. (Courtesy of the author)

without rigid structures or outside constraints. A more linear, reductive approach cannot capture the full complexity possible through such meanderings, but instead it can address only symptoms and not underlying causes. Despite the needs for quick fixes and strict accountability, danger lurks within highly structured forms of psychotherapy, with scripted forms of psychotherapy snuffing out spontaneity of all sorts. Too much reliance on formulaic or evidence-based approaches can rob therapists of opportunities to nurture imagination and intuition in a safe, open-ended playground.

The following case illustrates the continuity between early play and later life passions as facilitated through long-term, open-ended psychotherapy.

RALPH'S SHOOT-'EM-UP PLAY

The joys of conducting psychotherapy include seeing through windows into worlds into which we otherwise would have no access. The privilege of working with Ralph for over a decade was a case in point. As a young child, Ralph recalled endless imagination games he played with the neighborhood kids, all nearly the same age. Sometimes the boys played Cops and Robbers. Other times the game was Army or Cowboys and Indians. Whichever team he found himself on, Ralph was always passionate about the game and was usually the one who got shot and killed by the end.

These dynamics were notable in light of Ralph's family life. Whereas Ralph was the biological child of his parents, his younger brother was adopted. Ralph represented the calm before the storm of his brother's arrival several years later, when all chaos broke loose. Ralph's brother appeared to suffer pre- and postnatal damage from a drug-addicted mother. He was hyperactive, aggressive, and impulsive. Over time, Ralph's brother became a juvenile delinquent who later hardened into a criminal in and out of jail during much of his early adulthood.

Despite their huge differences, the two brothers got along reasonably well and had a loving mother who spent most of her emotional energy anguishing over her second child. Ralph's mother did everything she could to address her adopted son's problems, trotting the boy from one professional and facility to another. Nothing seemed to help. The stress on everyone was intense, with the entire family system organized around the drama. When Ralph was 8, his father had the first of his manic-depressive episodes, which became increasingly severe over time. When Ralph was a teenager, his mother developed ovarian cancer and then died within a few years.

Ralph adored and admired his self-sacrificing mother while feeling only disgust and contempt for his ineffectual father. Early on, Ralph learned to emulate the ways of his mother, a devout Catholic who always strove to be "good" by being compliant and suppressing all needs and feelings for the benefit of others. Ralph was particularly motivated to stamp out all signs of his father's powerlessness and anger by turning off negative feelings and cutting off awareness of burdensome needs that might drain the meager family resources.

Much as with Carl described earlier, we can see in Ralph's childhood play the whole of his family life. The "shoot-'em-up" games recreated the central issue of the family's never-ending fight with Ralph's brother. The neighborhood games provided a safe, titrated way to partake in and master the violence that was tearing his family apart. Ralph's emotional self-sacrifice at home was concretely enacted through being singled out by the neighborhood kids as the one to die for the benefit of the game. Meanwhile, Ralph's flip-flop between playing the good guy and playing the bad guy enabled him to remain empathic to his brother and to his parents at the same time.

I bring up this case partly to illustrate the diagnostic value of examining patients' early play experiences. These can provide clinical intuition with a bird's-eye view of passions, involvements, concerns, and lifelong preoccupations, not to mention occupations. Indeed, the flips in perspective available through childhood play also enabled Ralph to experience the psyche from both sides of the law. This continued to serve Ralph well in his professional life as an FBI undercover agent. Whether playing the role of a crooked apartment manager in cahoots with a neighborhood gang, a small-time drug dealer in search of a new stash, or a homosexual pedophile traveling abroad for young prey, Ralph had a highly nuanced view of his work. He prided himself on understanding the criminal mind and felt safe in relationship to his intuitive understanding, even when instructed to bring dangerous criminals right up to the edge of violence in order to be caught on tape.

Ralph's sophistication emerged at least partly because his professional intuition developed in the context of his early play experiences. Meanwhile, out of attachment and empathy for his brother, he could both infiltrate and remain compassionate with the criminal mind. Finally, in line with his early socialization, Ralph became a team player among agents, driven as much by compassion for others as by passion for his own work. Not once did Ralph allow ambition to compromise these prosocial values.

Ralph entered psychotherapy when he began to have panic attacks in the middle of the night, which started after the anniversary of a serious break-up. My clinical work with Ralph consisted largely in helping him to become aware of and express his inner feelings, especially fear and anger, while trusting his inner guidance and impulses. Clinical intuition is merely an offshoot of ordinary intuition that represents a healthy and necessary foundation for our being, doing, and relating in the world. When all goes well, there is beautiful continuity from early play to adult passions. Just as we therapists are healthiest when we can tap into and trust our intuitive side, the same holds for our patients. As therapists, part of the task of leading with intuition is to model this stance as a foundational position in life. The more we are grounded in our natural instincts, the more we can take in, absorb, and respond to outside information in a manner that is aligned with the whole of who we are.

THE REALM OF INSPIRATION

In keeping with this chapter's metaphor of intersubjectivity as a spatial and geographical coordinate system extending through time, I envision clinical intuition to be a *realm* of deep contact. When I enter this realm, I leave the solid shores of ordinary existence to navigate strange waters, where, if I am able to stay afloat, I sometimes serve as a vessel for a wind that seems to pass through me. To feel moved like this is to feel inspired, and inspiration is a key aspect of clinical intuition.

With regards to inspiration, I would like to share a story recently relayed to me by George, whose story of suppressed emotion and stifled creativity appeared in the last chapter. Recently George mustered up his courage to return to his creative writing. One evening, George took a break to attend a concert of improvisational world music with his wife. The musicians had not played together before. They decided to discuss their experience after they finished riffing together. One musician, whose usual manner of approaching performance was to be well prepared and well rehearsed, felt entirely uncomfortable in this *unfamiliar territory*, although he enjoyed the challenges of its discomforts. Another performer, whose career revolved regularly around improvisation, described himself as living for those *peak* moments of spontaneous creation when the musicians blend together into something utterly unique and nonreproducible.

This latter performer continued the discussion by analyzing the origins of the word *inspiration* to involve the act of taking in *breath* or *spirit*. In Hebrew, the word for "inspiration" is the same as that for "spirit." But in order to let the spirit move through us, we must be empty first, much like a flute must be hollow and empty in order for each breath to form its notes anew. When moved by the spirit of inspiration, then a reversal can take place, where the instrument becomes the musician and the musician becomes the instrument.

What a lovely image this was to me, especially given that emotion lies at the base both of inspired music and of psychotherapy! Meanwhile, so, too, does a similar reversal take place between the therapist and patient during psychotherapy. When in the throes of clinical intuition, when truly inspired by our work, there is often full interpenetration between the self and other, such that our patients *move* us while we *move* our patients. Spontaneous exchanges of emotion, energy, and information become forms of improvisation, including pulsating rhythms of call and response, synchrony, harmony, and counterpoint. When inspired in this way, the whole of me feels unified and deeply connected with the whole of the other. The mind, body, and soul get transported into unchartered waters by winds whistling through intuitive channels. And all the while, there is trust that no matter how perilous the journey, no matter what we may find, it is safe to journey there together.

WRAP-UP

The reader will recall from the last chapter the introduction of the delightful word *fingerspitzengefühl*, which literally means to have an intuitive sense of knowing at the tip of your finger. This "fingertip feeling" is not unlike our expression in English to "have one's finger on the pulse" of things. In both German and English expressions, intuition clearly begins with the body's capacity to move, sense, and feel. In this chapter, I join a multitude of others who have placed the body at the center of the feel of clinical work. I presented neurobiological evidence concerning the hippocampus that links the orientation of rats in physical space to the orientation of humans in social space. In both kinds of space, coordination and calibration of emotional, sensory, cognitive, and imagistic processes occur by "feel," through body-based feedback.

Just as rats need to explore physical space from all angles, so, too, must children have the freedom to explore social space from every angle of imagination. Only by becoming oriented from the inside out, by enfolding outer reality into the exuberances of inner fantasy games, do children become equipped to later navigate a path through life based on the solid foundation of intuition as aligned with the whole of themselves. According to this formulation, the dangers of overstructuring a young child's social environment become obvious. Too much structure can rob possibilities for imaginative play.

Similar danger appears to exist within highly structured forms of psychotherapy, where too much reliance on formulaic or evidence-based approaches threatens to rob our spontaneity and creativity. Upon open waters, where intuition is the ship, inspiration the wind, and deliberation the sailor, we therapists stand the best chance of successful encounters through clear perception and grounded response. Yet the meaning of a successful encounter will differ for each person and therapeutic dyad in each moment according to ever-shifting intersubjective currents. In order to bring the chapter's themes home to you and your clinical practice, please consider the following:

- If you were to imagine clinical intuition as a realm, how might you envision that realm? Does a picture come up, a feeling, a memory, or a set of words?
- Is this place metaphorical or physical for you?
- Is it a realm of feeling, doing, being, thinking, or relating?

- Is it a realm that feels tame and domesticated, or is it wild and unruly?
- Does this territory vary from patient to patient or does it feel consistent?
- Recall a time you felt *lost* with a patient. How did you find your way again? How did the adventure turn out?
- Now recall a time you felt moved by a patient. What does it mean to you to *feel moved* this way?

Next, in an effort to place clinical intuition within its fullest context for self-expression, we turn to the final chapter on wisdom.

CHAPTER 8

In Pursuit of Wisdom

The doors of wisdom are never shut.

—Benjamin Franklin

Men are wise in proportion not to their experience, but to their capacity for experience.

—James Boswell

Never does nature say one thing and wisdom another.

—Juvenal

PSYCHOTHERAPY DANCES AROUND DOMAINS OF BEAUTY, truth, and goodness. There is beauty in finding meaning and pattern and insight, even amid great suffering. There is emotional truth to be found in the eyes, hearts, and minds of every person. There is goodness in taking a "right action" that is ethical, true to the self, and dedicated to others' well-being. On a moment-to-moment basis, through clinical intuition, we discover these three values and juggle among them, sometimes consciously, more often unconsciously. While in the heat of the clinical moment, we continually draw on intuition as we choose how to attend, what to amplify, and what to ignore. Wisdom is the fruit borne out of years of listening to this intuition. To make such choices wisely represents our full flowering as practitioners. Therefore, it seems quite appropriate, if not necessary, for us not to leave the topic of intuition and psychotherapy without exploring the august place of wisdom in the arena of psychotherapy practice.

The topic of wisdom has intrigued thinkers in the humanities since antiquity. Yet only recently has the construct been operationalized by psychology researchers. A literature review by Meeks and Jeste (2009) within a PubMed database with "wisdom" as the keyword revealed a seven-fold increase in articles on this topic from the 1970s through 2008. Yet the total number was shockingly low—approximately 20 papers at the beginning of the time frame of the study and 150 papers toward the end. Meanwhile, within professional circles, the topic of wisdom is neither a standard aspect of clinical training nor a regular part of professional dialogue.

In an article appearing in an *American Psychologist* issue that was dedicated to positive psychology, Baltes and Staudinger (2000) defined wisdom as expertise concerning the "fundamental pragmatics of life." Pragmatics include understanding and judgment about the meaning and conduct of life, orchestration of human development toward excellence, and simultaneous attention to personal and collective well-being. I would guess that the majority of psychotherapists hold values in accordance with this set of pragmatics. Few of us enter the field to get rich. Most aspire to provide excellent service by helping patients improve the quality of their lives. Many have tasted the joys of serving others as a means to feed our own souls. I believe that when they operate in line with the highest values, the wisest therapists continue to blossom alongside patients.

I suggest that wisdom involves the fullest maturation of intuition, by which we navigate our physical and social worlds on a moment-to-moment and year-to-year basis. The more emotion, energy, and information that pours in from the outside, the greater the importance of a solid internal foundation from which to swim through the sensations, feelings, and facts while navigating sound choices. Because intuition depends on implicit knowledge drawn from a context, a solid internal foundation can only build over time, on the basis of a broad range of experiences, which is where wisdom comes in. Beginning therapists often launch their careers with exquisitely attuned sensibilities, but the most highly empathic people also run the risk of the greatest burnout and resonant trauma (Oakley, Knafo, Madhavan, & Wilson, 2011). True wisdom involves a balance between self- and other-care.

Although it is not an explicit focus, the recognition of wisdom is implicit in the mentor model of clinical training. By placing ourselves near highly esteemed, seasoned therapists, by watching how they respond, by hearing their war stories, by daring to share our deepest struggles and vulnerabilities, we create opportunities to watch and learn from their attention to intuition, and to absorb their wisdom by osmosis. Whether at the beginning of professional life or decades into practice, we all derive benefits from basking in relationships with evolved others. The mentor model is an age-old means to transmit wisdom through intuitive channels. Yet the time seems ripe to elevate the topic of wisdom to a more deliberate, conscious focus; that is the purpose of this chapter.

I admit that I am daunted, if not humbled, by my own ambitions here. Who am I to address the lofty topic of wisdom? Why should I proclaim my own clinical work worthy of this lens? After all, as Mahatma Gandhi said, "It is unwise to be too sure of one's own wisdom. It is healthy to be reminded that the strongest might weaken and the wisest might err." Despite self-doubt, I jump in anyway, inspired by a Latin phrase that rings in my "third ear" (Reik's [1983] phrase for clinical intuition): *sapere aude*.

Originally uttered by Horace, the motto "sapere aude" commonly graces educational and other civic institutions the world over (see Figure 8.1). The phrase translates loosely as "be bold, have daring, and take risks in order to gain wisdom." In later philosophical writings, the phrase was picked up by Immanuel Kant and Michel Foucault, with the aim of delivering the moral to a story about a naïve fool who waits for the stream to stop before daring to cross. Certainly this metaphor applies to the daily travails of clinical work. As we tackle messy, untamed, scary, seemingly unsolvable territories of people's troubles, there is value in the very endeavor itself, in efforts to gird ourselves up for the struggle, to wade through all that arises, to persist toward the light; in short, we muster whatever effort is needed to overcome often invisible obstacles.

In this chapter, I assert that wisdom in the clinical domain is two-fold. One dimension relates to excellence in self-care, and the other to excellent care of others. The true action lies in the balance and interplay between these two. After introducing philosophical foundations in the next section, I shift to wisdom in self-care. Once again I offer an animal story to indicate that even in the "highest" domains of moral sensibilities and ethical behavior, animals have much to teach us. Then I switch to the second prong: wise care of others. I return to Gus's case, first introduced in Chapter 2, to illustrate the following: A wise therapist tolerates ambiguity when not enough information is present. A wise therapist holds paradox gracefully when too much information bombards us. A wise therapist considers multiple frames of reference simultaneously, and he or she fluidly shifts focus from tiny details to huge events. A wise therapist skillfully oscillates between relevant events from the patient's past, relational unfolding in the room, salient aspects of present circumstances, and possibilities for an enhanced future. In short, a wise therapist holds in the background the widest possible perspective in which to place pieces of ongoing experience.

THE WISDOM OF INSECURITY

Within the practice of psychotherapy, it is important to distinguish between realms of knowledge, intuition, and wisdom. Whereas *knowledge* represents the accumulation and application of facts about our field *in*

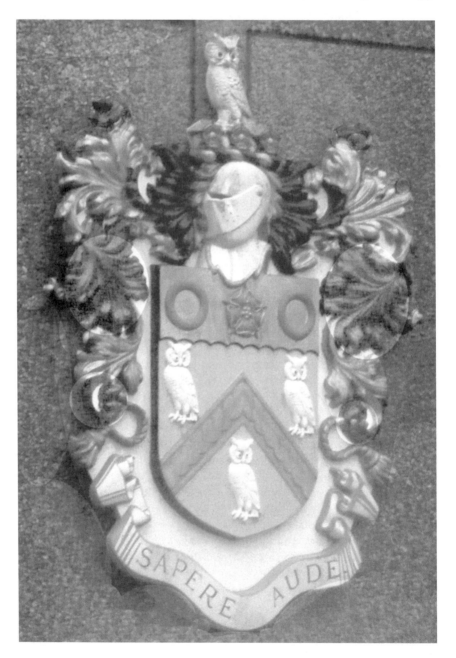

Figure 8.1. The phrase "sapere aude" translates loosely as "dare to be wise," and it appears here in Oldham County, Kentucky, in a coat of arms displayed on the Oldham Police Station building. (Public Domain.)

theory, intuition represents the accumulation and application of knowledge and expertise *in context*. Whereas *intuition* applies knowledge within the living framework of a real relationship with a real person in a particular moment, *wisdom* represents the capacity to use the *widest and deepest context* when making moment-to-moment assessments, decisions, responses, and interventions. Philosophy is one place where these distinctions are readily discernible, and, little wonder, as the origins of the word itself come from the Greek "philo-sophia," or "love of wisdom" (see Figure 8.2).

As I bumbled toward adulthood during the 1970s, I stumbled into a pillar of wisdom within the work of Alan Watts, a cultural "ambassador" and scholar who came from the West in order to gather pearls of philosophical wisdom from the East. In the preface to *The Wisdom of Insecurity* (1958), Watts described his earlier books as efforts to "vindicate certain principles of religion, philosophy and metaphysics by reinterpreting them." Watts likened this endeavor to "putting legs on a snake—unnecessary and confusing." By contrast, *The Wisdom of Insecurity* was written in the spirit of the Chinese sage Lao-Tzu: "To know truth, one must get rid of knowledge, and nothing is more powerful and creative than emptiness—from which men shrink."

Embodied in life, this philosophy translates to a *"warrior stance"* within psychotherapy (Coburn, 2011; Marks-Tarlow, 2011). The phrase derives from martial arts, where a warrior may train long and hard ahead of time, only to stand in inner quiet and outer stillness in the heat of the moment, in order to remain alert and ready for whatever may come. I believe great power exists in the warrior stance as it translates clinically to the embrace of uncertainty. During psychotherapy, this means *not having to know that which cannot yet be known*. To adopt this mental attitude allows us to remain emotionally open, cognitively poised and spiritually strong enough to withstand the heat of intense emotion, confusion, even delusion in our patients, not to mention ourselves.

A warrior stance permits encounters *at the edges* of the window of affect tolerance (Ogden et al., 2006; Siegel, 1999) in arousal zones that are "safe, but not too safe" (Bromberg, 2006), *without having to know* what will happen next. When working with high-intensity arousal, a not-knowing stance helps us to stay afloat in charged conditions of ambiguity, contradiction, or conflict. Under lower levels of arousal, a warrior stance cultivates curiosity, play, and creativity by maximizing openness, a desire to learn, and receptivity to novel input.

In a previous paper, "The Certainty of Uncertainty" (Marks-Tarlow, 2003), I examined how ancient Chinese wisdom dovetails with the non-linear science of chaos theory, partly by comparing the two as creation myths. Traditional creation myths, both Eastern and Western in origin, present static tales that speculate about the origins and nature of the

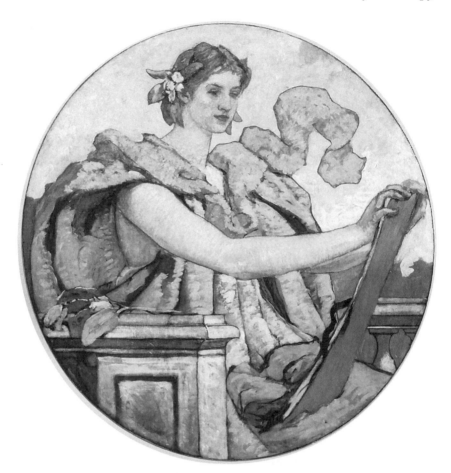

Figure 8.2. *"Wisdom"* by Robert Lewis Reid, 1896. Inspired by Sophia, the Goddess of Wisdom, this mural appears on the second floor of the North Corridor of the Library of Congress, inside the Thomas Jefferson Building in Washington, DC. The caption underneath reads "KNOWLEDGE COMES *BVT* WISDOM LINGERS." (Public domain, courtesy of Carol Highsmith)

universe. Science, both in linear and nonlinear forms, represents a special kind of creation myth that is dynamic and continually evolving through an open, ongoing dialogue with nature. Ancient Chinese wisdom and nonlinear science share the common features of embracing ambiguity and paradox in their understanding of the universe and its creative origins.

Whereas folk psychology collects the wisdom of individuals, creation myths collect the wisdom of cultures. When the highest wisdom strikes a universal chord, then the implicit knowledge of ancient peoples sometimes is borne out later by scientific proof (see Figure 8.3). This occurred with chaos theory, where the wisdom of the warrior (i.e., the wisdom of insecurity) presaged limits to predictability and control discovered within highly nonlinear systems (e.g., Gleick, 1987). According to chaos theory, no matter how much we understand about the current and even past states of a complex system, we remain doomed to fail at predicting future states, especially in the long term.

Within psychotherapy, this means that no matter how well we know our patients—how much we understand the origins of their problems, the complexity of their issues, the uniqueness of their being and plight—we can never be certain exactly where they are headed or what will happen in the future. In fact, a warrior stance suggests it is a waste of time trying to predict too precisely. Much like the flute waiting to be inspired by the breath, warriors empty their minds in order not to waste mental energy. Part of the challenge of psychotherapy is facing the terror of the unknown. We get distracted if we calculate endless lists of "what-ifs," most of which will never come to pass. We remain much more firmly planted to deal with actualities as they arise if we relax into the self-trust of sensing, risking, and hoping that we are prepared for *whatever does happen*. This helps us to tolerate not knowing until the moment when we actually do know.

This mental stance can be extremely difficult, especially for beginning therapists. Without a wealth of previous experience by which to gauge their own terror, it becomes difficult for therapists to sense what is happening at the boundary between the self and other. Here is a clinical example. A student in a recent class presented a case of an 8-year-old, highly depressed boy, who was inactive and mute to the point of scaring the therapist. While the patient was not overtly suicidal, this highly attuned therapist feared for the boy's life. The student's preoccupation and worry continued until one day, when the fledgling therapist brought one of her young patient's dreams into her psychoanalytically oriented supervisor. Being seasoned and comfortable within this population, the supervisor could point to hidden strengths that were evident in subtle aspects of the child's dream. This greatly reassured the student, allowing her to relax into the work. The ability to make such judgments accurately requires a wise supervisor who can place current information within the wider context of other such dreams as they have emerged from other such emotional states. Again, this is only possible over time, with lots of experience. Such context-dependent, context-sensitive knowing differs greatly from the facts of knowledge as systematically taught, *even if the content is identical*.

To better understand the difference between knowledge and wisdom, it helps to compare creation myths of the West with those of the East (including traditional cultures everywhere). The prototypical Western myth displays black-and-white thinking. The brave knight kills the scary dragon as pictured in Figure 8.4a. Good overcomes evil. Order vanquishes chaos.

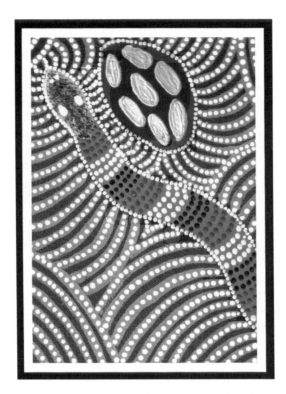

Figure 8.3. This detailed portion of an Aboriginal dot painting by Pixie Brown is from the collection of the clinical psychologist Jan Berlin. When contemplating intuition within the broadest context of wisdom, consider the roles of culture and mythology to mold experience and shape ideals. Some cultures are more naturally intuitive than others. Because the Aborigines live in one of the harshest environments on Earth and have a deep sense of interconnectedness with all beings, their culture is highly intuitive. The practice of psychotherapy can draw on this notion of interconnectedness to tap into wisdom through attunement, mutuality, and the cultural appreciation for each client's individual story. This piece depicts an Aboriginal creation story. The snake represents Kuniya, the Python Woman, who carried her eggs to Uluru (a giant monolith in Central Australia that is highly revered by the Aboriginal people). Kuniya, a powerful protectress, was eventually transformed into the Rainbow Serpent, a central figure in Aboriginal cosmology. The wavy lines symbolize both the tracks that Kuniya made when she searched for food and the energetic patterns that are believed to vibrate with song all over the earth. A wise therapist embraces meanings and honors traditions arising from different eras and areas, celebrating all sources of diversity, whether ethnic, genetic, gender-based, or skill-driven.

The story is simple and straightforward. Chaos must be eliminated in order for civilized society to begin or advance (Hayles, 1990). Strict dichotomies set the stage for left-brain, reason-based thinking, including modern, scientific investigation as grounded in Aristotelian logic (true or false).

Western creation myths point toward the following characteristics of left-brain thinking:

- Linear: lines of thought follow *sequential reasoning*;
- Abstract: issues are *abstracted from context*;
- Convergent: attention *focuses in on details*;
- Analytic: complex issues are *pulled apart logically*; and
- Reductive: wholes are *broken down into simpler* underlying parts.

By contrast, Eastern and traditional creation myths highlight dynamic, swirling, ambiguous zones in between the black and white. In these myths, chaos and order are interdependent and interpenetrating. The prototypical Chinese dragon may be scary and intimidating, but shades of gray are revealed by the dragon that ultimately cooperates to enrich humankind. The dragon may guard pearls of wisdom in the sky, as pictured in Figure 8.4b. Or the dragon might live in clouds to create thunder, lightning, and rain for crops, or it may be in the fields to dig moats with its mighty tail.

Eastern myths point to right-brain modes of thinking with the following traits:

- Nonlinear: reasoning is *cyclic or circular*, including polarities that blend or contradict;
- Concrete: issues are *lived in context*;
- Divergent: attention *broadens out* to encompass a wide angle view;
- Synthetic: understanding emerges from the *complex inter-relationship* among simpler parts; and
- Holistic: complex understanding arises from *how the whole of things informs and forms the parts*.

We easily visualize complex, fully interpenetrating realms of dark and light within the yin-yang symbol as shown in Figure 8.5. Conceived as a circle, not a line, only together do the parts compose a whole, with the seeds of each planted within holes in the center of the other. An even more complex, infinitely recursive version is formed when the inner circle is replaced by a tiny version of the other side.

In a previous book (Marks-Tarlow, 2008a), I explored the interface between Eastern wisdom and nonlinear science as it applies to clinical practice. The branches of nonlinear science that are relevant to clinical

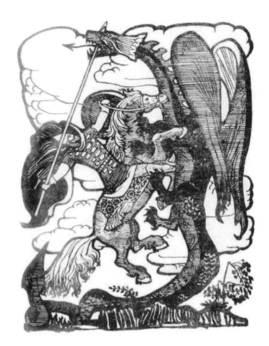

(a)

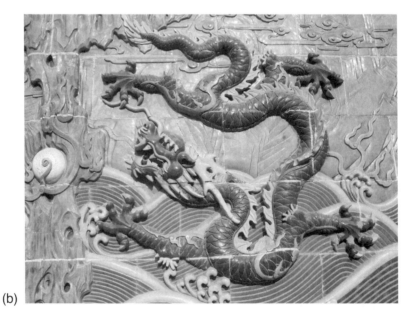

(b)

Figure 8.4.   (a) Order vanquishing chaos in a Western creation myth;
(b) Chaos and order intermixing in a Chinese creation myth.

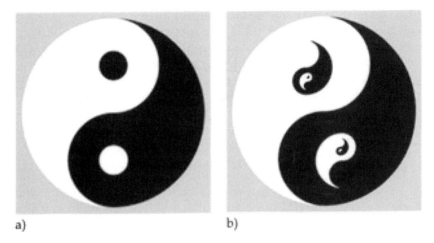

a)   b)

Figure 8.5. (a) Traditional and (b) recursive forms of the yin-yang symbol. According to ancient Chinese thought, yin and yang represent opposite forces in nature as they swirl dynamically and partially interpenetrate. Yin is dark, downward moving, cold, passive, contractive, and weak; yang is bright, active, upward moving, warm, expanding, and strong. Yin symbolizes clinical intuition, as it originates in and emerges from the invisible or dark unconscious, while yang represents conscious deliberation as it emanates from the clear light of reason and known fact. (Courtesy of the author)

practice include chaos theory, fuzzy logic, complexity theory, and fractal geometry. Chaos theory illuminates limits to certain knowledge and the futility of trying to predict exactly where people or relationships are going, especially during unstable times of crisis or transition. Fuzzy logic offers multivalent systems (many values besides true and false) of logic that apply readily to realms of emotion and the unconscious. Complexity theory reveals complicated, novel structure as it emerges unpredictably from intersubjective bases. Finally, fractal geometry uncovers the recursive, recurrent patterns of nature, especially found at the edges of highly complex systems. Within psychotherapy, fractals model the messy, entangled boundaries between the self, the world, and the other.

The myths of the East complement those of the West by giving rise to nonoverlapping realms of understanding. In the spirit of McGilchrist (2009), it is useful to contrast two modes of knowing: a linear realm available through left-brain deliberation and a nonlinear realm available through right-brain intuition. Just as there is a place for both modes in the full tapestry of world mythology and accompanying culture, so, too, there is a place for both modes during the enterprise of psychotherapy. One way to understand wisdom is as the very practical skill of shifting between these two modes of perceiving, knowing, and investigating in the most effective, pragmatic manner possible. With this philosophy in mind, let us shift back to some neurobiological roots of wisdom: our human ethics, by which we intuit and care about justice and fairness in relationships with others and ourselves.

THE PLAY OF JUSTICE

In Chapter 3, I examined the roots of clinical intuition within the mammalian care system. Given that we birth immature infants who are completely dependent on others for survival, it is critical that we have the capacity to understand the minds of others in order to respond to the babies' needs. In *Braintrust,* the philosopher Patricia Churchland (2011) likewise traced the roots of human moral intuition to the mammalian care circuit. Here, the motivation to nurture and help others blends in with the desire to *be ethical* and *do the right thing*, as more general aspects of social intelligence. Here, too, these higher qualities spring from subcortical capacities that Homo sapiens share with other "social animals."

While it is not surprising that humans share primitive emotional states like rage and fear with lower animals, it may seem more surprising that we also share more evolved sensibilities, including a sense of justice and fairness. The more closely we observe all animals, especially in their natural habitats, the more even the "lower" ones appear to do amazing and sophisticated things in service of self- or other-care. Bees communicate the whereabouts of food to hive mates through complex wiggle dances. Mice stop feeding themselves in response to witnessing pain administered to a cage mate, though not to a stranger. Elephants sometimes bury their dead, and they are driven by remarkable memories to recognize more than 200 fellow herd members. Bottlenose dolphins can make tools by breaking off pieces of sponges to protect their noses while foraging for food. Gorillas make calculations by using walking sticks to measure the depths of rivers they wish to cross. Chimps adopt human symbols by learning sign language or by using the computer for purposes of interspecies communication (see Figure 8.6).

Naturalistic studies reveal that all mammals who live in large social groups display a code of ethics. What is more, tendencies to treat others in a just and fair manner are most easily detectable during play. Once again, we see that play is serious business. In a 2004 paper entitled "Wild Justice and Fair Play: Cooperation, Forgiveness, and Morality in Animals," Marc Bekoff argued that studying social play among group-living animals helps us to understand the evolutionary origins of social morality. Bekoff believed that evolution strongly selects for cooperative fair play. This enables individuals

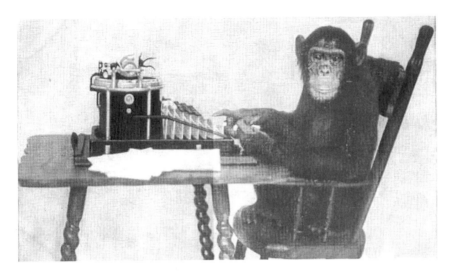

Figure 8.6. Although this chimpanzee at a Yost typewriter could not actually produce a meaningful text on this type of old-fashioned machine, chimps nowadays are quite adept at using computers to communicate with people in strings of symbols. The controversy is no longer whether chimps can use human language, but instead it has moved to whether chimps can use grammar when communicating with humans. (Produced by the New York Zoological Society, 1907)

to establish and maintain social contracts that maximize their chances to survive and propagate while simultaneously stabilizing the group.

In a more recent book, Bekoff and Pierce (2009) indicated how animals within the dog family, or canids, play ethically according to four key rules:

1. *Communicate clearly*: Canids announce their intentions to play, rather than fight, with partners, by employing a ritualized play bow as the consistent invitation for fun. They crouch on their forelimbs while standing on their hind legs. Notice the similarity of this position to the downward-facing dog pose in yoga (see Figure 8.7). This humbling posture allows us to meet the ground with all four limbs, inviting heavy thoughts to drop out of the top of the head through gravity.
2. *Mind your manners*: Canids consider their partners' feelings and abilities. For example, a coyote might refrain from biting a playmate too hard in order to self-handicap and keep things fair. Or a dominant pack member might perform a role reversal by rolling

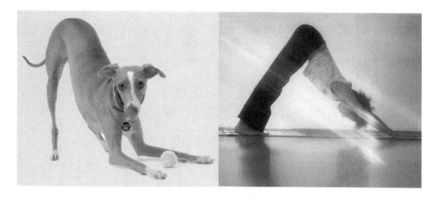

Figure 8.7.   (a) Dog making a play bow; (b) Woman doing a downward-facing dog pose. (8.7a © Margaret Bryant Photography; 8.7b   Courtesy of Jeanne Heileman)

over on her back to signal submission, a gesture that would never happen during real aggression.

3. *Admit when you are wrong*: If play gets out of hand, and an animal accidently hurts a partner, an apology is forthcoming. For example, after a bite that is too hard, the offending animal bows as if to communicate, "Sorry, I only meant to play; I didn't intend to hurt you. Please don't leave. I'll play fair." The animal's partner must forgive the transgression in order for play to begin anew. Forgiveness happens most of the time, during play as well as in daily pack life, where understanding and tolerance are usually forthcoming.

4. *Be honest*: When apologies are made, they must be sincere. Animals that continue to play unfairly or send dishonest signals inevitably get ostracized. According to Bekoff's field research, juvenile coyotes forced to leave the pack are up to four times more likely to die than those that remain inside.

These key rules amount to guidelines for addressing emotional rupture and repair during animal play. Within clinical psychology theory, rupture and repair is a broad, central tenet to emotional growth (e.g., Lewis, 2000; Schore, 2003a) in patients. Especially when early relational trauma is high, clinical lore suggests that we therapists inevitably trigger upsets for patients that are similar to disruptions with early caregivers. This opens up opportunities for the therapeutic pair to forge a different outcome from the traumatic variety experienced previously. New structure builds as therapists carefully empathize with their patients' perspectives, no matter how much these perspectives may differ. In this way, therapists can take responsibility for their role in triggering or fueling the patients' upset. To take responsibility in this way often means to apologize for insensitivities and mistakes that are made. A wise therapist is one who can empathize and apologize humbly, with grace. By modeling compassionate, nondefensive engagement around upset and conflict, therapists can help build patients' capacity to keep the needs, feelings, and perspectives of two people in mind *simultaneously*—the essence of intersubjectivity.

Bekoff's animal research revealed how the rupture-and-repair sequence, as performed during play, complements the rupture-and-repair sequence emerging out of the caring circuit to soothe newborn distress. Fair play represents an important way that mammals extend positive intentions and just behavior beyond the immediate family. This would suggest that impulses to repair upset and resolve interpersonal conflict are not just qualities of those who have a "big heart." Instead they also indicate capacities for sound ethics and just treatment emerging quite literally from "fair play." To recognize this helps us to understand more about therapist motivation, specifically why it feels so important to provide good care across the board, even to patients whom we may not particularly like.

This rupture-and-repair sequence constitutes the "corrective emotional experience" that Franz Alexander (Alexander, 1961; Alexander & French, 1946) proposed so long ago as the cornerstone of relational healing. How interesting, if not leveling, that the same sequence can be detected within the fair play of animals, which may even represent its evolutionary origins at the societal level. Along with a means for exercising neural plasticity, the play circuit evolved hand in hand with the care circuit as a vital way to extend fair behavior throughout the social community. Meanwhile, it appears that even with the lofty topic of moral behavior, we find animal precursors to fair and compassionate action. Whether involving communication, self-awareness, empathic resonance, tool use, or, now, ethical behavior, each capacity has been erected as the definitive line between humans and animals, only to be torn down again.

WISDOM: A TWO-PRONGED AFFAIR

Within the clinical domain, I have proposed wisdom as a two-pronged affair. One prong involves the excellent treatment of others. As we saw above, this appears clearly to be the case among social animals and is largely derived from the instincts to care for young and weak group members as well as to play fairly. The other prong involves excellent care of the self. What does fair treatment of others have to do with good treatment of self? This brings to mind a story I heard about the Dalai Lama, considered a pillar of wisdom by Tibetan Buddhists (e.g., Dalai Lama, 2010). When

His Holiness first came to the United States as a young man, the Dalai Lama was utterly shocked and dismayed by the degree of self-loathing he encountered. Not only had he never seen this phenomenon before, but he actually had a hard time understanding it culturally. Apparently, among Tibetan Buddhists there is no distinction between compassion for others and compassion for the self. Because they go hand in hand, there is no separate concept for the two. Wisdom suggests that the capacity to care for and honor the self is absolutely vital to the capacity to care for and honor others (see Figure 8.8). We saw through the example of play that animals possess a sense of justice, fairness, and compassion for one another. What about the self-care component of wisdom—do animals share this as well? The section to follow offers a resounding "yes."

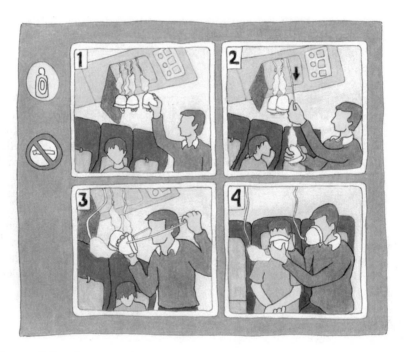

Figure 8.8. Anyone who possesses doubts about what comes first— self-care or other-care—should study this image carefully. The drawing is fashioned after instruction cards that are routinely available in the seat pockets of all airline seats. In the case of oxygen failure, this card instructs all passengers to put on their own oxygen masks before attempting to assist anyone else, including small children, to put on theirs. Many basic truths start with body wisdom. (Courtesy of the author)

Horse Sense in Self-Care

The *Collins English Dictionary* defines "horse sense" both as "common sense" and "sound practical judgment." In order to demonstrate how horses can have sound practical judgment as relates to self- and other-care, I offer an animal tale from my childhood when, like so many other little girls, I loved horses. Each summer I was sent to a girls' sleepaway camp in Maine for two months. As the years went by, I started spending more and more time at the stables, until I reached the point of relentlessly begging my parents for a horse. They resisted.

"We aren't a 'horsey' family," my mother replied. "No one in our family rides, or knows anything about horses, including how to take care of them. Besides what makes you think you have talent with horses anyway?" (As the reader might detect, my mother was rather elitist.)

Needless to say I didn't get a horse at that point. However, I did manage to convince my parents the following summer to let me switch from an all-round camp to sleepaway horse camp in Vermont. Each girl was assigned to ride and take care of her own horse for the entire session. Initially, I was disappointed in the horse assigned to me. As is apparent by name alone, Chunky was not skinny and she was not pretty or flashy. But she sure was old. In fact, at 24 years of age, Chunky was almost ancient for a horse. Yet I was so grateful just to be at horse camp at all that I quickly resolved to make the best of it.

As the summer progressed, I could not have been more thrilled by what happened. After much training and riding, both in the ring and on the trails, the summer culminated in everyone entering a local riding competition. Out of all the campers, I was the only one to win a ribbon, receiving second place in a hunter/jumper class. With this impressive showing under my belt, I subsequently won the award for Best Rider at the end of the summer. While the thrill was dampened by knowing in my heart that Chunky deserved the award much more than I, I nonetheless trotted home happily, ribbon in hand. For now I had the evidence I needed to prove to my parents that I *did* have talent in the horse arena.

The plan worked. That fall, my parents bought me a horse—a 4-year-old chestnut thoroughbred named Tickertape, previously owned by a stockbroker. I was in heaven. I wanted to ride as often as possible. Yet, immediately, a huge problem emerged. Every time I mounted Tickertape, I splattered to the ground. At times, my spirited horse could buck or rear me off from a standstill. Fortunately, for me, my parents were not "horsey" people. They would drop me off at the stable and pick me up at the end of the day without learning what happened in between. Had they known, I suspect they would have taken Tickertape away. While I suffered lots of bruises that first year, not the least of which was to my pride, I am happy to say I stuck it out. Within a few years, I actually became a good rider. To this day, despite my somewhat ripened age, I retain the confidence to get on any horse without fear.

Looking back, I owe my foray into riding completely to Chunky's wisdom. I really was right about that award from camp. I had not been a good rider, but instead I had been lucky to be assigned to a mature horse who knew how to take excellent care both of herself and of me. Being old, vulnerable, and wise, Chunky could pace herself perfectly when approaching a jump. This was the sole reason that I placed high in the hunter/jumper competition. Chunky truly loved to jump. All I had to do was to point her in the right direction and stay on top. Despite my being a lousy rider and unable to guide her properly, Chunky was a wise horse with ample ability to guide me instead. Thus, in taking care of herself she was also taking care of me.

Wisdom in the Body

The story of Chunky reveals wisdom partly as a function of age. Age certainly plays a part in people's implicit theories of wisdom (Bluck & Glück, 2005). Young horses can be wild and reckless. Subject to whim and passion, they easily hurt themselves. Stories abound of prideful horses doing anything to break out of unwanted enclosures or of overly ambitious horses attempting jumps beyond their capabilities. Older horses are much more likely to refuse unwise choices, for example, by stopping short of an inappropriate jump or shying to the side at the last moment. Even for horses, horse sense develops over time, with experience.

Beginning psychotherapists often are quite skilled out of the gate, due to their natural empathy or informative early life experiences. Yet because wisdom becomes internalized on the basis of experience, only seasoned clinicians can be wise. Studies of expertise reveal what has been termed "the 10-year, 10,000-hour rule" (Gladwell, 2008; Obler & Fein, 1988). That is, it takes *either* 10 years *or* 10,000 hours of practice in order to gain full competency in any skilled enterprise. This holds as true for mastery in chess as it does for mastery on the viola, in musical composition, cooking, dance, science, or virtually any other area of the humanities, arts, or sciences. We now understand how the 10-year, 10,000-hour rule works. Because full mastery in a complex skill depends on the implicit rather than explicit domain, it takes that amount of time for underlying neural circuitry to establish the necessary foundation to embrace any future possibility. In other words, after 10,000 hours or 10 years, people have sampled the full range of variability as it relates to the skill in question. This then permits full integration, efficiency, and complexity.

Within the realm of psychotherapy, while I began clinical practice with fairly good instincts, I, too, noticed a definite shift in my sensibilities approximately 10 years into my work, about which I have written previously

(Marks-Tarlow, 2008a). Ironically, the biggest difference involved my attitude toward *what I did not know*. That I did not know everything I needed or wanted to know was no longer a signal to me of my own deficiency or lack of professional knowledge. Rather, I stopped squirming so much about information I did not yet possess. I began to recognize this feeling of uncertainty as normal—the existential lay of the clinical land. This has allowed me to feel more emotionally regulated and less panicked when I didn't know what's happening or how to respond.

There is an old British saying, "Knowledge is proud because She knows so much; wisdom is humble because She understands so little." Within the clinical domain, wisdom and humility definitely go hand in hand. Wisdom arises in the fuzzy, dark, uncertain, intuitive realms associated with right-brain flashes and hunches, while knowledge is collected in the sharper, crisper, brighter, and more certain sensibilities of left-brain thinking. The relationship between these two faculties represents a never-ending flirtation of yin with yang, safety with danger.

While the story of Chunky suggests that age, or at least extended experience, is a necessary ingredient for wisdom, this does not mean age or experience guarantees the full flowering of intuition into wisdom. In fact, whereas the implicit theories often associate age with wisdom, empirical studies reveal a more complicated relationship between these variables (Sternberg & Jordon, 2005). But if there is no guarantee of wisdom with age, what else is needed? Returning to Chunky's story, this horse matured so well precisely because she understood her body thoroughly, including its limitations. When it came to navigating through a world of obstacles, including inexperienced child riders, it was Chunky's relationship to her own body—her form of self-care—that provided her horse sense.

I believe the same thing translates over to psychotherapy. In this realm, self-care involves care of our own bodies, minds, and spirits in the context of relationships. Along with leading a balanced life by feeding, exercising, and resting our bodies, this includes attending to our limits and boundaries, and extending compassion to our selves through emotional understanding and self-knowledge. Without this embodied piece, age and experience bring no guarantees of expertise. Without this embodied piece, we run the risk of burnout, compassion fatigue, and the inability to sustain enthusiasm and maintain natural gifts over the long haul. Within clinical practice, the deepest wisdom emerges out of the fullest capacity to utilize the totality of who we are. In order to care for others well, we must be able to read not just with our minds but also with our bodies; also, we must be able to respond not just to others but also to ourselves. This requires an understanding of how emotions, gut feelings, hunches, and inspirations—in a word, "intuitions"—all manifest within our particular physiology. What is more, we must continue to read the impact of our bodies' presence in the world. This feedback dimension is critical.

As a yoga teacher as well as a clinical psychologist, I love sending patients to yoga in order to draw parallels between the practices of yoga and psychotherapy. I find this so valuable because yoga is a system of embodied progress. After being personally immersed in yoga practice for 30 years, I have probably stepped onto my own mat 10,000 times. Every time I do, there is only one thing I hope for—that it will bring new experience in some form. I have come to recognize variation in how my body/mind/brain feels on my mat, ranging at one pole from a thin, almost tinny experience of shallowness where I am rushing my way through, hoping to get somewhere, but never arriving; at the other end is a rich depth of experience, a complex interfolding, where I am aware of multiple layers to savor, and the slower I move through the better.

I stated above that yoga provides an embodied model of progress. But what is progress, really? Especially in our culture, it is easy to think of progress as bettering and perfecting ourselves. In life, this can amount to a relentless, if not ruthless, search for perfectionism. In yoga, this can translate to an emphasis on physicality and trick poses, such as the one pictured in Figure 8.9. But I prefer a more literal, embodied sense of the word—*progress as progression*, a dynamic flow and unfolding over time that happens naturally. By bringing our entire past to bear, each encounter with

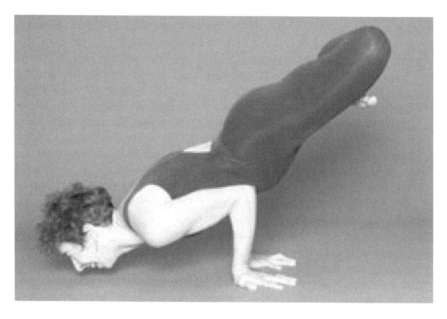

Figure 8.9. Who said an old yogini can't learn new tricks? This photo was part of a shoot taken to celebrate my 53rd birthday. (Courtesy of Victoria Davis Photography)

the mat becomes a new opportunity, if only for rest or restoration. We can attend to the dynamics of the moment as they lay enfolded in the shifting dynamics of our current states and developmental stage.

When we are young, we become caught up in the natural exuberance of our bodies' physicality. As we age, we fold in transcendence as offered by the body's spirituality. Ideally, at all stages of life and all states of being, the challenge of each moment is to seek a balance between determination and surrender, strength and flexibility. This balance leads to moments of *effortless effort*. These states emerge from the cessation of doing for attainment; instead, doing unfolds intuitively and naturally from the center of being. Here, the pure joy of expression regularly touches the pleasure of play. Simply by showing up for practice, attending to alignment, coordinating movement with breath, and fully immersing ourselves in the process, we are nearly guaranteed changes in our bodies, minds, and spirits. By setting intentions at the beginning of each session to guide our focus and concentration, and by receiving adjustments along the way by experienced teachers, we are bound to improve our strength, flexibility, balance, focus, and coordination simply by remaining fully engaged in the practice itself.

Within the practice of yoga, to be wise means to honor the idiosyncrasies of our own bodies as the material sheath for the rest of who we are. Each time we step onto the mat, it is a new experience. Our bodies are different, and so are our minds. It does not serve us to compete with anyone else, or even with our own performance from a previous time. One day we might feel energetic and raring to go. The next day we are gripped with fatigue or fighting off a cold. On certain days we might be filled with sadness. Each condition affects our body differently (Fogel, 2009; Ogden et al., 2006). Each condition requires a different response. When we are energetic, we may feel open to trying new, challenging, or scary poses. When our bodies feel weak, we need to back away from physicality and seek restorative poses and resting states. When we are sad, we might want to nurture our vulnerability by meditating and connecting with our spiritual centers. In each case, the "edge" we seek is different.

The Sanskrit word for wisdom as earned through deep practice and experience is *vidya*. *Vidya* allows us to sink under fogged perceptions and ignorance to the place where clear sight and deep connection are possible—to others, to the source of being, to our true self. So, too, during psychotherapy, wisdom brings the grace of self-reflection amid greater nuance. A wise therapist knows and supports the fullness of his or her own self, inside and outside, attending accordingly. Without this and other forms of self-care, we cannot be present or available to others. Within psychotherapy, self-care has a variety of meanings. In a single moment, it means paying attention to how we feel as we enter sessions with patients, and honoring that information as a foundation for attending to the other.

In the larger view, it means doing our very best to embody the work of psychotherapy ourselves. Just as we expect priests and religious figures to uphold higher moral values, therapists ideally aspire toward wisdom by fostering a keen self-knowledge, maintaining excellent relationships, and leading exemplary lives. Returning to Lakoff and Johnson's (1980) primary set of metaphors, to embody our own work entails seeking an *upright posture* and a *balanced stance* in life. Along with value-driven, ethical behavior, this might include good nutrition, regular exercise, and broad pursuits of self-expression. Along with filling our lives with meaning and meaningful relationships, exemplary living also means knowing when to reach out for help from others, whether consultants, supervisors, doctors, or, of course, psychotherapists.

WHOLES IN THE HOLES

Having covered the first prong of therapeutic wisdom, excellent care of the self, I now turn to the second prong: excellent care of others. This wisdom embodies the important qualities of tolerating ambiguity, fusing opposites, holding complexity, and not knowing. In order to illustrate these essential characteristics, I wish to immerse the reader in Gus's clinical case, drawing heavily on a previous write-up (Marks-Tarlow, 2011). Recall from Chapter 2 that Gus was the 62-year-old man who contacted me for help to rid himself of his experience of feeling like a woman at times. Here is some background to the joys and discomforts of sporadically feeling female, which began when Gus was 36, surrounding the breakup of his first marriage, 15 years into the relationship.

Gus had hit a limit to feeling unappreciated, burnt out, and "used" for the material support he provided. Unable to talk to his wife directly about extreme hurt and growing resentment, Gus enacted his distress instead. This followed a poignant discussion on a ski lift near their second, mountain house. Gus's wife mentioned her desire to acquire yet a third house on the beach. Gus began doubting his wife's love for him apart from what he provided. He soon tested his theory unconsciously by imploding his own business. Unfortunately, Gus was right; his wife left him. In the decades that followed, Gus suffered a series of other relationships characterized by similar emotional themes of exploitation and emotional neglect.

The pattern appeared to break with Gus's second wife, who clearly loved him despite his ongoing struggles with money. Yet Gus still had difficulty communicating about emotions and other significant aspects of his inner life. Increasingly, he took refuge in the female part of himself. Here Gus was safe to feel his feelings, while complete isolation from others (not to mention from his own male aspects) alleviated all pressures to communicate.

Upon entering psychotherapy, Gus also had not recovered from his work trauma. After his divorce, along with other difficult relationships, he continued on a downward spiral professionally. Incident after incident brought Gus still lower. He was fired as CEO of a business after suffering a heart attack. He lost significant amounts of money, as well as his best friend, after a business they started together failed. When Gus first came to see me, he was underemployed, underpaid, and incredibly frustrated with his rigid, at times floridly schizophrenic, boss.

While I am comfortable with highly diverse populations in the Los Angeles area, I had never encountered anyone quite like Gus. Despite this lack of familiarity, from the start of treatment, quite unconsciously, I adopted a warrior stance. That is, I tried to steady myself in my own discomfort surrounding not knowing. Rather than seeking counsel from others or reading up on the literature, I stood firmly in the intimacy of our budding relationship. I trusted that everything I needed to know would emerge in its own way and in its own time. (Mind you, I had nearly 30 years of practice under my belt. I do not recommend here that people step beyond the bounds of their own competencies!)

Indeed, this was a trial by fire, as my trust in fully immersing myself in the unknown was tested over and over. One way was discussed previously, when initially Gus's "symptom" worsened rather than lessened. Another way involved many unexpected occurrences in Gus's life as his therapy progressed. One dimension of this involved Gus's relationship to his music. Along with his sexual fantasies, for many years, Gus also used to take solace in composing music. In the last chapter, I described synesthesia in Gus's eventual relationship with his music, where this realm of expression became so available to him that he could shed his body, figuratively speaking, and enter the music as an auditory space with physical extension.

Yet at the point of starting therapy, Gus had not written a song for 12 years. His last piece—inspired by his father's death and conceived with the help of marijuana—concerned the theme of death. The song, written for solo voice without accompanying instrumentation, had been sung aloud only once, in a darkened recording studio, with Gus's back to the technicians. No one had heard the song because Gus could not bear the pain of hearing it.

After much talk about the link between leaving his music along with other pieces of himself he wanted to eliminate, Gus readied himself to play his music as part of our therapy. The process took months. As we got closer, Gus would bring the CD player into my office. There, it sat alongside the two of us for weeks until the time felt just right. When that moment occurred, Gus played several other compositions first, winding up with the last song he had written. This was the song that ended all songs, partly because it was "so perfect" in Gus's mind, that he could not imagine topping it. This led Gus to wonder why he should bother to write anything else.

Upon hearing Gus's song, I was struck by how emotion-filled I felt. Yet it was difficult to put words to my strange and poignant mixture of feelings. It was as if fragments of feelings led me away from the center, where the music hinted at a hurt so deep that it could only be buried. I noted the intense emotionality of the lyrics, including thoughts about anesthetizing one's self so as not to feel pain yet knowing the pain was still there. I was especially chilled by how the song ended—with a long, unpredictable, and arrhythmic gap between two words: "quiet" and "home." Later, I would learn that during the recording of the song, Gus had actually dissociated between those two words and that was the reason for the gap and its erratic nature.

During the next session, we continued processing our listening together. Gus shared the following dream.

> *I am pregnant. I arrive at the hospital with my husband, but then he drops away from the scene, and I don't see him again. I am being wheeled by a nurse down a long hall toward the delivery room. As they prep me for delivery, I begin to protest, "I don't know how to do this! I've never done this before! I'm afraid of screwing it all up." The nurse responds by reassuring me. Over and over she says, "You'll be just fine. We'll get through this together."*

Gus and I examined parallels between bringing in the dream and playing me the song. Both involved facing dark and fertile holes of the great unknown. Both included potentially bottomless pits of pain, without knowing what would come of it. Yet in both cases, someone was there to say, "Don't worry, I'm with you. It will all be okay." The pain of listening, coupled with Gus's desire to feel his way into how his music had entered me emotionally, opened up our discussions tremendously. We broke new ground concerning Gus's lack of emotional safety, including all the gaping wounds and holes in Gus's emotional life.

The song's theme of the death from war highlighted Gus's internal war with himself—with his feminine side, plus the recursive twist of being at war with his own war. This inner (k)not appeared more like *a void*, in line with Gus's implicit rule always to *a-void* the war of conflicted feelings. Over the next several weeks and months, we returned again and again to transference dimensions apparent from Gus's dream of me-as-nurse wheeling him down a corridor into the unknown where he attempted to birth and rebirth parts of himself. As we focused on what Gus was trying to "conceive" within himself, a poignant moment of meeting occurred when, in a highly vulnerable moment, Gus shared his longing for me to serve as the midwife to his music.

The Music Under the Words

Not long after all of this, Gus learned that his 19-year-old, unmarried administrative assistant, Tina, was pregnant. The young woman immediately went into crisis about whether or not to keep the baby. Gus became the sole voice of encouragement in this woman's life, a stance that related at least partly to his own history. Gus's mother had been abandoned by her husband during her pregnancy. Later Gus's mother met a loving man who adopted Gus. Gus had always experienced his adopted father as his "real" father. Curiously, the pattern was repeating intergenerationally, because Gus's current wife also had a child by another man. Like his own mother, Gus's second wife was abandoned by the father of her child. When Gus came on board, that child was 3 years old. Gus came to feel about his second wife's child the way his adopted father felt toward him. In fact, 18 years later, Gus now felt closer to his adopted son than to his biological daughter from his first marriage.

With all this history behind him, Gus became Tina's close confidante, as he supported and encouraged her through her initial crisis surrounding an unplanned pregnancy. The two grew extremely intimate emotionally. The closer Gus felt to Tina, the more Gus's experience of his own female side merged with that of his administrative assistant. In fact, Gus was in lock-step alongside Tina through the various stages and sensations of pregnancy. Gus's somatic experience was so physiologically grounded that the young woman was surprised at Gus's ability to anticipate her embodied experience. One night as Tina approached delivery, Gus had a dream:

> *Tina is about to deliver her baby. She's all alone. Her mother is angry with her for choosing to have the baby. She won't help. Tina comes into my office and asks me to be her Lamaze coach. "Of course!" I reply without hesitation or much thought, even though I know deep down in my heart that my wife would later protest my decision.*

Gus's administrative assistant's pregnancy became the inspiration for Gus's heart to spring open, such that during "their" respective pregnancies, Gus reclaimed his music. Without the help of marijuana, Gus heard a love song, written as if from a mother to a newborn. But as Gus described the song, I heard a double meaning. I imagined an unconscious expression of love written as if from Gus to the young woman. Meanwhile the more Gus talked during our sessions about his caring for his administrative assistant and her baby, the stronger his determination became no longer to be a "prisoner of fear"—too scared to support the stirrings of his heart. The stronger Gus's determination grew to express his feelings, the more uncomfortable and scared I began to feel about what was going on.

Everything felt precarious and ominous, as if slipping toward disaster. I was the one with a war inside of me now, as I struggled to balance such wildly mixed feelings. On the one hand, I experienced joy in Gus's emotional opening along with his reconnection with his music. I intuitively knew Gus's music came from his female side and this brought him ever closer to integration. Yet I struggled with intensely negative feelings at the same time. Gus's preoccupation with his love song combined with his

Lamaze dream revealing motives quite apart from his wife's feelings, and this caused me to bristle. I sensed great danger to his marriage. An image was triggered in my mind of a train racing downhill, off its tracks, about to crash into old, repetitive patterns of implosion and explosion. And to top it off, I felt deeply divided about what portion, if any, of my mixed emotions to share with Gus.

All of this prepared the way for one session in particular that felt like an electrifying "moment of meeting." Gus began with the following risky observation.

"There's something I need to check out with you. I've noticed a subtle shift in you lately. A couple of months ago, whenever I brought up the subject of Tina, you would squirm a bit in your chair. You would change position; your posture would stiffen; your voice would get thin and strained; your words became clipped. But, now, that no longer seems to be the case. You appear much more comfortable with me when the subject of Tina comes up. Is this all so?"

Gus's observations about "the music under the words" stunned me at first by calling attention to aspects of myself about which I had been mostly unaware. I took a moment to self-reflect. Then, after carefully investigating Gus's fantasies about my inner relational world and its meaning to Gus's own sense of self, safety, and well-being, I chose to reveal the picture as seen from my side of the couch.

"What you say is all true, Gus. I was thoroughly uncomfortable about what was happening. I was delighted in your openings yet scared it would all come to a screeching halt if you acted on your love instead of holding it inside to serve as a source of inspiration. I wanted to say something to you. I wanted to warn you of my fears, but I held back. I didn't want to shame you and, besides, I knew you had to find your own truths.

"But now, as you call all of this to my attention, I realize how far my experience *has* shifted. I've stopped worrying. I feel at ease again. I guess I've come to a position of trust that you can hold the full complexity of your experience, without needing to implode inside or to blow your marriage to bits. The 'danger' seems to have passed."

Within a couple of weeks of this seminal session, despite his mature age and years of job seeking, Gus landed a high-level executive job. Gus got the position by using the same intuitively penetrating skills he had used with me during our moment of meeting. First, he had accessed the website of the job site. Then, he had analyzed it scrupulously to identify strengths and weaknesses in the business. Finally, he created a fancy PowerPoint presentation, including a plan surrounding his visions for the business. When he made his presentation, Gus used his highly perceptive read on the members of the board, all of whom were part of one family. The group was unanimously floored by Gus's intelligent discernment and almost psychic abilities to diagnose the contours of their business. Not only was he hired, but he also was given full license to take the small business in any direction he envisioned (and all while earning approximately three times his former salary).

HONORING TWISTS AND TURNS

As wise therapists, we serve as midwives to the creation of wholeness in our patients. Those of us who are privileged enough to be engaged in long-term psychotherapy with patients in hopes of deep transformation know firsthand that no matter how much we clean and polish the fruits of our teaching stories or case presentations, the process is always messier than our sanitized versions of linear narrative streams. This is where knowledge has limited value, intuition is essential, and wisdom is so inspiring. As I have written previously "To truly enter into the relational dance means to surrender to its fits and jerks, to cultivate the patience necessary to sometimes grind to a standstill, to close our eyes metaphorically, while we allow ourselves to grope, glide and sometimes leap by feel alone; and always, always throughout, to adopt a warrior's stance of not having to know what is coming next" (2011, p. 115).

In response to a lack of emotional safety, Gus both rejected and simultaneously yearned for split-off aspects of his self. Before he started psychotherapy, Gus feared he had to be rid of the fantasy of himself as a woman in order to be potent as a man. Over time, through increasing feelings of safety, he came to understand the opposite: Gus's very attempt to give up pieces of himself in hopes of preserving relationships with others was itself leading to feelings of impotency, implosion, and burnout. Only by reclaiming these split-off pieces could Gus feel powerful and whole. We also came to understand Gus's concrete experiences of himself as a woman partly in symbolic terms, as reflecting conflicting impulses to dissociate unbearable feelings while yearning for a connection to his feeling side along with the rich internal life it afforded him. Finally, at the level of the underlying neurobiological dimension, Gus's symptom appeared to be a left-brain, logical mind dissociated from and in search of a right-brain, emotional, relational side.

EMOTION AS THE MUSIC OF INTEGRATION

Another aspect of therapeutic wisdom illustrated in this case is how Gus intuitively guided and taught me about himself and myself, much as Chunky did so many years ago. This part of the case illustrates the wisdom within the intersubjectivity of our respective intuitions.

Although Gus was initially uncomfortable with the language of dissociation, when we discussed his transition away from stress and into his female side, he eventually found this formulation useful and descriptive. Gus moved past his shock at the possibility of having dissociative identity disorder, and this relatively new way of describing a multiple personality disorder eventually became most befitting of Gus's actual experience. In fact, here is a description Gus gave of his own subjective experience one day.

"It's a paradox. I dissociate because I don't want to feel. But when I dissociate, it becomes all about emotion. This is because, as a woman, I enjoy what I feel."

"What an interesting observation!"

"I think I can explain the paradox. As Gus, when I feel the urge to dissociate, it's because I'm feeling something negative, something uncomfortable. But, as a woman, it's all good. I'm not Gus any longer; he fades into the background as someone else who feels all that negative emotion."

"What about when you go into the music? That sounds different yet again."

"Yes, when I go into the music, it is different. There, it's not all positive feeling at all. There's a whole landscape of dynamic action. The territory is filled with emotions that I can sense but can't always name—that is, until later, when I can look back and say, 'Oh, that's what that was!' "

"Your music seems to act like a bridge between Gus and his emotions."

"Somehow emotions are safer in the music. I can hate what I'm feeling, but if I love the music, it becomes easier to deal with the cognitive dissonance."

"And what does that feel like?"

"I leave my body. Everything is black. All is sound. I enter into the music and the notes, and *that* is all there is. Then I work out the song. *Only later do I realize that I'm working out my emotions as well.* Because I love the music, I can settle the dissonance of not liking the feelings, which are now wrapped in love. Sometimes I actually feel the feelings as I come out of the music; other times, I work out that part later.

"The music is like an exoskeleton of the body I enter when mine disappears. When I wrote my last song, I really needed to disappear. Here was my wife saying, 'Don't touch my things, don't touch my life, but why don't you jump into bed with me right now and touch my body.' I did it, but emotionally it was too much. I had to leave. So I left and went into my musical world. A new song immediately came to me. It was so compelling. I've never heard anything like it. The music began mechanically, like a clock that beats time." He beats his hand on the couch loudly and rhythmically.

"'Mechanical' is the same word you used for how you pleasured your wife."

"Yes, but after just two measures, it changed to the string section, where it was soft and vulnerable, crying out for more."

"That's how you have been feeling in relationship to your wife—at least up until recently when it's been striking you that she may not have more to give."

"And then the music changed again, but I wasn't able to finish it in bed. When I was done pleasuring her, I got out of bed. I went to the keyboard, but I couldn't hear the ending. I kept trying to force it, saying to myself, 'It sounds classical; what would Beethoven do here?' But that didn't work."

"Just like trying to force a certain resolution with your wife hasn't worked either."

"So after a couple of days of this, I just let go and then literally went back into the music. I let *it take me* where it needed to go."

"That's how emotions (not to mention intuitions) work for most of us. Especially when we trust them, they take us where they need us to go."

"So then I heard the next section as a bridge back to the beginning, mechanical part. Except this time it was different; it was slower, as if the journey to get back there took a lot out of me."

Throughout our years of psychotherapy together, Gus's perceptiveness has continued to amaze me. I have felt awed at his ability to tune into nuance, both inside himself and inside of me. Part of my amazement involves a circular sense that Gus's focus and perceptiveness enhances my own clinical capabilities. It is likely that I selected this case for a chapter on wisdom precisely because of these qualities within him. If I have been a wise therapist in this case, it has been primarily because Gus was a wise patient. Consider the words of Walter Lippman: "It requires wisdom to understand wisdom: the music is nothing if the audience is deaf." Just as the horse taught the rider in Chunky's case, so, too, did the patient elevate the therapist in Gus's case.

Whoever first invented the cliché "you can't teach an old dog new tricks" failed to consider how experience can temper and ripen the body through time. Perhaps wisdom that comes with the embodied understanding of age is one factor that helps patients be more open and receptive to psychotherapy later in life. Certainly this concurs with recent neurobiological evidence that people can retain certain faculties into old age, especially as our brains retain a fair degree of neuroplasticity throughout life (Siegel, 2007, 2010).

THE MATERNAL WISDOM IN US ALL

In order to illustrate Gus's capacity for body wisdom and positive change, I present one more moment of meeting between us. Again the discussion was initiated by Gus, who called attention to a gap he noticed in my communication in the prior session. We had been discussing a highly emotional encounter between Gus and his son. After the boy turned 18 and no longer needed a signature from his biological father (with whom he had no contact), he requested that Gus legally adopt him. Gus happily assented. In preparation, Gus's son also decided to drop his own last name, which belonged to his biological father, and adopt Gus's last name instead. When the boy's mother (who had yet a different last name from both) heard of her son's intentions, she became furious. Upon learning of his mother's fury, the boy "broke down" emotionally. First the boy expressed anger by hitting a wall with his fist, and then he dissolved into tears. For many minutes, Gus held his son tenderly in his arms as he cried.

After hearing this account and feeling quite moved, I uttered, "That was very motherly of you," only to then awkwardly add, "and fatherly as well. . . ."

The next week, Gus opened the session with "I want to go back to something you said last week. Do you remember I was telling you about holding my son while he sobbed and you said, 'That was a very motherly thing to do'? Then there was a slight pause. Your voice changed, and you added, 'It's fatherly as well. . . .'"

"How did my voice change?"

"It got more strained, almost hesitant, as if caught in your throat. . . . Here is my question: What happened during that pause?"

"Okay, good question. Give me a moment. . . . [long pause] I think I got uncomfortable about what I had said. That comment about your being 'motherly' came out so spontaneously and naturally. But then, after blurting it out, I *heard* what I said."

"What do you mean?"

"I think I added 'fatherly' for fear that if I attributed motherly qualities to you, this might feel like an insult. But that wasn't the only thing. I'm also guessing I added 'fatherly' for my own benefit. I didn't want to sound sexist. I didn't want to think that only women held their children that way when they feel distressed. To be honest, I'm not sure how much I added 'fatherly' for your sake versus my own. But either way, it was definitely an afterthought—a deliberate, almost forced addition."

"Hmm . . . yes, I definitely sensed your discomfort. But I want to tell you something important to me. I *wasn't* insulted *at all*. In fact, I took what you said as a compliment. I like being thought of as motherly."

"I think I sensed that it would be okay when the words first flew out of my mouth."

"And there is something more I've realized recently that I also need to talk about. There's been a change in me over the last couple of weeks. I feel different inside. I have a much greater comfort than before. This is because *She* is always there now.

"Really?" I inquired. I could feel my eyebrows rising with interest. "Tell me more."

"Do you remember how it was before? Gus was always there; *She* came out only now and then. Whenever *She* was out, Gus remained aware, but he was in the background. Yet the reverse was not the case—*She* was never aware of Gus."

"Sure, I remember that well."

"Now it's different. Both *She* and Gus are always present. At times *She* stays in the background and Gus enters the foreground. At other times it's the reverse. But now it's never 100% one way or the other. It's always both. I don't know how to explain this." Gus gestured with his hands. They were stretched out straight in front, side by side. As one hand moved forward, the other pulled back closer toward his body. Then he switched which hand was forward and which was back, repeating the gesture a couple of times.

"I get it," I replied. "Your hands tell the story. It's like a figure/ground switch that reminds me of the eye's fovea. As one thing comes into sharp focus, everything else blurs to the background, until the focus switches yet again. But the other thing I realize from your description is that you no longer have energy invested in keeping *Her* away."

"Exactly! I feel *completely* comfortable with *Her* now. *She's* there and *She's* not going anywhere. This brings us full circle to the beginning of our work together. On the phone, you said that in all likelihood, it would not be possible for me to rid myself of *Her*."

"At that point in time you hated *Her*. Now it appears that you love *Her*."

"I *do* love *Her*. I see and feel how much she brings to my life!"

EMBRACING COMPLEXITY

What is mental health, if not the freedom to feel every nuance of emotion, without judgment, whether positive or negative? What is wisdom, if not the capacity to hold complexity, by embracing the entire range of feelings, both in the self and other? Whether you are a therapist or patient, to hold the wisdom of full complexity is to protect yourself from imploding in self-destructive ways or exploding in relationship-destructive ways. Much of the complexity in Gus's case can be found in the space between implicit and explicit levels. From the very first contact by phone, Gus asked me over and over to "penetrate him" with a diagnosis in service of "emptying" his yearning to be a woman. But at the implicit level, the relational dynamics were more complex. Gus needed me to be a midwife rather than to rape or abort his primary experience.

The wise therapist knows when to penetrate with understanding and when to receive and hold emotion with compassion, switching between modes intuitively as necessary. The wise patient allows in both masculine and feminine aspects with androgynous freedom, especially as our dominant culture moves further away from preset, prescribed sex roles. Such relational patterns were enfolded recursively within Gus's history of music making and his dreams. With me as the nurse to his pain and the midwife for his emotional expression, a greater ability to reconnect with his unique inner voice, greater creativity, and greater integration were possible. Integration also included the capacity to penetrate my body language and receive and contain my implicit emotional expression. The wise therapist knows how to be inspired and guided by the natural wisdom that exists within our patients. The notion of mutual interpenetration within the intersubjective field supports such concepts, partly by positing a self that is fully enfolded within the other while the other is fully enfolded within the self, much like the yin-yang symbol depicted in Figure 8.5. With clinical intuition, therapists can tap into the infinite expanses and inseparability of these dynamics.

Fusing Opposites

Meeks and Jeste's (2009) review article on the neurobiology of wisdom observed that brain areas that underlie wisdom contain both the evolutionarily oldest and the newest structures among mammals. Old areas include the hypothalamus, brain stem, and amygdala; newer areas include the cingulate and prefrontal cortices. There is something lovely about the full circle of wisdom encompassing both the old and the new. How reminiscent of the wisdom of the ages as it passes on from one generation to the next, as transmitted from elders to youth. This circle of wisdom is also reminiscent of the Uroboros—the snake that swallows its own tail (Marks-Tarlow, Robertson, & Combs, 2002). Here, opposites come together, as the beginning fuses with the end of the snake in a literal, embodied way.

In myths the world over, the Uroboros symbolizes self-reflection, self-generation, and renewal. In ancient Egypt, the Uroboros is depicted on tombs as the guardian of the Underworld. It represents the liminal moment when death encounters resurrection. In the West African vodun religion of Benin, the Uroboros appears as an icon for the god of order, Dan. Dan mediates between the world of the gods and our world, in order to create order in the wind, water, and other cyclic, often chaotic, rhythms of nature. In old European maps (see Figure 8.10), the Uroboros swims among other mythological creatures in distant seas to symbolize the fearsome edges where the known meets the unknown.

In modern mathematical notation (e.g., Varela, 1975, 1979), the Uroboros represents form as it re-enters itself, creating time in the process. In psychology, re-entry involves the incorporation of feedback into processes that repeat over time, yet never do so exactly, as new end products serve as new beginnings for the next round. Whether through attuned response, error correction, or rupture-and-repair sequences, incorporating feedback enables us to adapt, learn, and change. The old informs the new while the new reforms the old. This capacity to integrate opposites in the service of flexible adaptation and response is how wisdom develops.

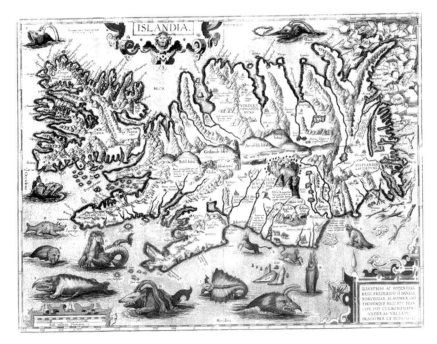

Figure 8.10. This map of Islandia (now Iceland) reveals the Uroboros and other creatures who inhabit the edges of the known. (Photo courtesy of Normal Thrower)

As therapists, we hold a metaphorical bag of tools that contains many pairs of opposites. At times we come forth; at other times we hold back. At time we insist; at other times we relent. At times we attend to content; at other times we disregard content in order to attend to process. At times we are active; at other times we are receptive. At times we disclose; at other times we withhold. At times we move frantically; at other times we are still. At times we guard our boundaries furiously; at other times we soften to make room for exceptions to rigid rules.

Round and round we go, cycling through opposite responses, often multiple times even within the course of a single session. Where do we place our attention? How do we bind these opposites? How do we find what is most emotionally salient within a sea of sensory impressions and cognitive facts? This is the realm of clinical intuition. To do so in a fashion that honors ever larger wholes is how integration occurs and where everyday clinical intuition morphs over time into wisdom. The Uroboros keeps eating its tail/tale, and if we are lucky, we grow ever wiser in the process. Wisdom refines clinical intuition to become our guide.

WRAP-UP

Knowledge is devoid of lived experience, while intuition and wisdom are both embedded in life. Knowledge can be accumulated rapidly; intuition is instantaneous; and wisdom requires time and patience. Whereas knowledge can be organized and staged, intuition and wisdom are spontaneous and inspired. Knowledge speaks of facts; intuition hints at the inner story; wisdom finds the point and the moral. Knowledge can be taught; intuition needs to be preserved; wisdom must be discovered. In the splendor of the psyche, wisdom sits high atop the paradox. Wisdom appears when we least expect it. No sooner do we grab for it than it disappears. Wisdom, like intuition, creativity, and other implicit processes, is ephemeral.

Elizabeth Gilbert (2009) described a personal story relayed to her by the poet Ruth Stone, now in her nineties. As Stone worked in the fields of rural Virginia, she would feel and hear a poem coming at her from over the landscape, "like a thunderous train of air barreling down at her," shaking the earth. At that point Stone knew there was just one thing to do—to "run like hell" to the house, while being chased by the poem. She had to get a paper and pencil fast enough so she could collect it on the page. But sometimes she would not be fast enough. She would miss the opportunity, and the poem would continue barreling down the landscape, looking for another poet. Once in a while, as it barreled through her, Stone would catch just the tail end of it. When this happened she would pull the poem back into her body as she transcribed it. At these times, the poem would come out transcribed backward, from the last word to the first.

The realm of therapeutic wisdom is similar. It may come through us but is not of us; within its realm, everything is backward. No sooner do we think we have arrived at wisdom than we lose our way. Perhaps, it is better to look at wisdom sideways, through the corner of our intuitive eye, without any claim to ownership. This preserves the humility that is so central to it. During a *Psychology Today* interview, Robert Sternberg, one of the few wisdom researchers, disavowed knowing anything much about the subject at all. Paradoxes such as these become poignant as we strive broadly toward goals that are impossible to reach. Here, the words of Theodore Roszak (in Marks-Tarlow et al., 2002, p. 20) are haunting: "The mind is gifted with the power of irrepressible self-transcendence. It is the greatest of all escape artists, constantly eluding its own efforts at self-comprehension."

When attempting to integrate the daunting topic of wisdom in psychotherapy, consider the following:

• Who are the wise therapists you know? What qualities do they have?

- How would you define wisdom as a therapist?
- What role does age versus experience play in achieving wisdom? Is it possible to be naturally wise? How universal versus tied to culture is the concept?
- Does your work and being embody your vision of a wise therapist? Have you achieved a nourishing balance between self- and other-care?
- How important to the therapeutic community at large is discussion and research about wisdom?

EPILOGUE

Healing within psychotherapy involves a search for wholeness, full engagement, and complexity in the present moment in the presence of another. Clinical intuition is the primary tool by which we psychotherapists feel our way through this process. Sometimes patients need to soften rigid edges, abandon worn-out defenses, breathe life into dead places, integrate disowned parts, or resist the pull of ancient habits that no longer serve them. Clinical intuition is the faculty of the mind/body/brain system by which we take stock of where we stand in intersubjective space. By informing us of relational patterns in the past and present, clinical intuition also serves as the creative conduit toward a different future. And because psychotherapy is a two-way street, the opening of intuitive faculties proves just as critical to patients for navigating life and filling it with meaning.

Whether we do so consciously or not, whether as a therapist or patient, each of us waits for those windows of intuitive inspiration when something unexpected and novel emerges without planning. These moments can take years of preparation and patience, but they are what successful therapy is all about. A new form of intimacy or contact, increased interest in one's own internal life, or the ability to self-regulate emotionally or behaviorally represents something different or important entering a patient's life. These gifts often emerge out of times when we feel inspired as therapists. To continue to feel inspired and nourished over time allows wisdom to emerge as the full flower of intuition. In the process, good psychotherapy can continue to emerge as the full flower of wisdom.

With this book, I aspire to bring the topic of clinical intuition to the forefront of therapists' consciousness. I realize it is only a beginning, but if nothing else, I hope this work helps to elevate clinical intuition as part of our neurobiological heritage as playful, caring, and wise animals.

References

Adolphs, R. (2003). Is the human amygdala specialized for processing social information? *Annals of the New York Academy of Sciences, 985*, 326–340.

Ainsworth, M., & Bowlby, J. (1965). *Child care and the growth of love.* London: Penguin Books.

Alexander, F. (1961). *The scope of psychoanalysis.* New York, NY: Basic Books.

Alexander, F., & French, T. (1946). *Psychoanalytic therapy: Principles and applications.* New York, NY: Ronald Press.

Allman, J.M., Watson, K.K., Tetreault, N.A., & Hakeem, A.Y. (2005). Intuition and autism: A possible role for Von Economo neurons. *Trends in Cognitive Sciences, 9*, 367–373.

Amos, T. (2006). *Piece by piece.* New York, NY: Broadway.

Andrade, J. (2009). What does doodling do? *Applied Cognitive Psychology, 24*, 100–106.

Arizmendi, T. (2008). Nonverbal communication in the context of dissociative processes. *Psychoanalytic Psychology, 25*(3), 443–457.

Badenoch, B. (2008). *Being a brain-wise therapist: A practical guide to interpersonal neurobiology.* New York, NY: W. W. Norton.

Baltes, P. B., & Staudinger, U. M. (2000). Wisdom: A metaheuristic (pragmatic) to orchestrate mind and virtue toward excellence. *American Psychologist, 55*, 122–136.

Barbas, H. (2007). Flow of information for emotions through temporal and orbitofrontal pathways. *Journal of Anatomy, 211*, 237–249.

Barrie, J. (1896/2011). *Margaret Ogilvy.* New York, NY: New York Public Library.

Bastick, T. (2003). *Intuition: Evaluating the construct and its impact on creative thinking.* Kingston, Jamaica: Stoneman & Lang.

Beatty, W., Dodge, L., Dodge, A., Dodge, L., White, K., & Panksepp, J. (1982). Psychomotor stimulants, social deprivation and play in juvenile rats, *Pharmacology, Biochemistry & Behavior, 16*, 417–422.

Beebe, B., & Sloate, F. (1982). Assessment and treatment of difficulties in mother-infant attunement in the first three years of life: A case history. *Psychoanalytic Inquiries, 1*, 601–623.

Beeman, M., Friedman, R., Grafman, J., Perez, E., Diamond, S., & Lindsay, M. (1994). Summation priming and coarse semantic coding in the right hemisphere. *Journal of Cognitive Neuroscience, 6*, 26–45.

Bekoff, M. (2004). Wild justice and fair play: Cooperation, forgiveness, and morality in animals. *Biology and Philosophy, 19*(4), 489–520.

Bekoff, M., & Pierce, J. (2009). *Wild justice, the moral life of animals.* Chicago, IL: University of Chicago Press.

Benner, P., Hooper-Kyriakidis, P., & Stannard, D. (1999). *Clinical wisdom and interventions in critical care.* Philadelphia, PA: W. B. Saunders.

Benner, P., & Tanner, C. (1987). Clinical judgment: How expert nurses use intuition. *American Journal of Nursing, 87*(1), 23–31.

Berkower, L. (1970). The military influence upon Freud's dynamic psychiatry. *American Journal of Psychiatry, 127*, 167–174.

Bion, W. (1967). *Second thoughts.* London: William Heinemann.

Blakemore, S., Wolpert, D., & Frith, C. (2000). Why can't you tickle yourself? *NeuroReport, 11*, 11–16.

Bluck, S., & Glück, J. (2005). From the inside out: People's implicit theories of wisdom. In Sternberg, R. & Jordon, J. (Eds.), *A handbook of wisdom: Psychological perspectives* (pp. 84–109). New York, NY: Cambridge University Press.

Bohart, A. (1999). Intuition and creativity in psychotherapy. *Journal of Constructivist Psychology, 12*, 287–311.

Bollas, C. (1987). *Shadow of the object: Psychoanalysis of the unthought known.* New York, NY: Columbia University Press.

Borins, M. (2003). Are you suffering from a laugh deficiency disorder? *Canadian Family Physician, 49*(6), 723.

Boucouvalas, M. (1997). Intuition: The concept and the experience. In R.D. Floyd & P.S. Arvidson (Eds.), *Intuition: The inside story* (pp. 39–56). New York: Routledge.

Bowlby, J. (1969). *Attachment* (Vol. 1). New York, NY: Basic Books.

Bowlby, J. (1973). *Separation: Anxiety & anger* (Vol. 2: Attachment and loss). International Psycho-Analytical Library No. 95. London: Hogarth Press.

Brokensha, G. (2002). Clinical intuition: More than rational? *Australian Prescriber, 25*(1), 14–15.

Bromberg, P. (2006). *Awakening the dreamer: Clinical journeys.* Mahwah, NJ: Analytic Press.

Bromberg, P. (2011). *The shadow of the tsunami and the growth of the relational mind.* New York: Routledge.

Brown, S. (1998). Play as an organizing principle: Clinical evidence and personal observations. In M. Bekoff & J. Byers (Eds.), *Animal play: Evolutionary, comparative and ecological perspectives* (pp. 243–259). New York, NY: Cambridge University Press.

Brown, S. (2009). *Play: How it shapes the brain, opens the imagination, and invigorates the soul.* New York, NY: Penguin Group.

Bucci, W. (2011). The interplay of subsymbolic and symbolic processes in psychoanalytic treatment: It takes two to tango—But who knows the steps, who's the leader? The choreography of the psychoanalytic interchange. *Psychoanalytic Dialogues, 21*, 45–54.

Bugelski, B., & Alampay, D. (1961). The role of frequency in developing perceptual sets. *Canadian Journal of Psychology, 15*, 205–211.

Bugental, J.F. (1987). *The art of the psychotherapist.* New York: W.W. Norton.

Burgoon, J. (1985), Nonverbal signals. In M. Knapp & C. Miller (Eds.), *Handbook of interpersonal communication* (pp. 344–390). Thousand Oaks, CA: Sage.

Burns, S., & Brainerd, C. (1979). Effects of constructive and dramatic play on perspective taking in very young children. *Developmental Psychology, 15*(5), 512–521.

Buzsáki, G. (2006). *Rhythms of the brain*. New York, NY: Oxford University Press.

Campbell, J. (1949/1973). *Hero with a thousand faces*. Princeton, NJ: Princeton University Press.

Charles, R. (2005). *Intuition, counseling and psychotherapy*. New York, NY: Wiley.

Churchland, P. (2011). *Braintrust: What neuroscience tells us about morality*. Princeton, NJ: Princeton University Press.

Cioffi, J. (1997). Heuristics, servants to intuition, in clinical decision making. *Journal of Advanced Nursing, 26*, 203–208.

Claxton, G. (1997). *Hare brain, tortoise mind: How intelligence increases when you think less*. New York, NY: Ecco Press.

Coburn, W. (2011). A warrior's stance: Commentary on paper by Terry Marks-Tarlow. *Psychoanalytic Dialogues, 21*, 128–139.

Cortina, M., & Liotti, G. (2007). New approaches to understanding unconscious processes: Implicit and explicit memory systems. *International Forum of Psychoanalysis, 16*, 204–212.

Coulson, S., & Wu, Y. (2005). Right hemisphere activation of joke-related information: An event-related brain potential study, *Journal of Cognitive Neuroscience, 17*(3), 494–506.

Cousins, N. (1979). *Anatomy of an illness as perceived by the patient: Reflections on healing and regeneration*. New York, NY: W. W. Norton.

Cozolino, L. (2005). *The neuroscience of human relationships: Attachment and the developing social brain*. New York, NY: W. W. Norton.

Csikszentmihalyi, M. (1990). *Flow: The psychology of optimal experience*. New York, NY: Harper and Row.

Csikszentmihalyi, M. (1996). *Creativity: Flow and the psychology of discovery and invention*. New York, NY: HarperCollins.

Cytowic, R. (1993). *The man who tasted shapes*. New York, NY: Tarcher.

Dalai Lama (2010). *The Dalai Lama's little book of wisdom*. Newburyport, MA: Hampton Roads.

Damasio, A. (1996). The somatic marker hypothesis and the possible functions of the prefrontal cortex, *Philosophical Transactions of the Royal Society of London, 351*, 1413–1420.

Damasio, A. (1999). *The feeling of what happens*. New York, NY: Harcourt Brace.

Darwin, C. (1872). *The expression of the emotions in man and animals*. London: John Murray.

Dawson, G., Webb, S., & McPartland, J. (2005). Understanding the nature of face processing impairment in autism: Insights from behavioral and electrophysiological studies. *Developmental Neuropsychology, 27*(3), 403–424.

Decety, J., & Ickes, W. (2009). The social neuroscience of empathy. Cambridge, MA: MIT Press.

Delignières, D., Fortes, M., & Ninot, G. (2004). The fractal dynamics of self-esteem and physical self. *Nonlinear Dynamics, Psychology, and Life Sciences, 8*(4), 479–510.

Dinger, U., Strack, M., Leichsenring, F., Wilmers, F. C., & Schauenberg, H. (2008). Therapist effects on outcome and alliance in inpatient psychotherapy. *Journal of Clinical Psychology, 64*(3), 344–354.

Doidge, N. (2007). *The brain that changes itself*. New York, NY: Penguin Books.

Dooley, L. (1941). The relation of humor to masochism. *Psychoanalytic Review, 28*, 37–48.

Dorpat, T.L. (2001). Primary process communication. *Psychoanalytic Inquiry, 3*, 448–463.

Dreyfus, H., & Dreyfus, S. (1986). Why computers may never think like people. *Technology Review, 89*(1), 42–61.

Eels, T. (2001). Attachment theory and psychotherapy research. *Journal of Psychotherapeutic Practice and Research, 10*, 132-135.

Effkin, J. (2001). Informational basis for expert intuition. *Journal of Advanced Nursing, 34*(2), 246–255.

Einon, D. (1980). Spatial memory and response strategies in rats: Age, sex and rearing differences in performance. *Quarterly Journal of Experimental Psychology, 32*, 473–489.

Eisenberg, N., & Strayer, J. (Eds.). (1987). *Empathy and its development*. New York, NY: Cambridge University Press.

Ekman, P. (Ed.). (2003). *Emotions inside out: 130 Years after Darwin's "The Expression of the Emotions in Man and Animals"* (1st ed.). New York, NY: New York Academy of Sciences.

Ellman, S. (2010). *When theories touch: A historical and theoretical integration of psychoanalytic thought*. London: Karnac Books.

Emde, R. (1983). The prerepresentational self and its affective core. *Psychoanalytic Study of the Child, 38*, 165–192.

Fabian, E. (1982). On the differentiated use of humor and joke in psychotherapy. *Psychoanalytic Review, 89*(3), 399–412.

Fisher, H. (1994). *Anatomy of love: A natural history of mating, marriage, and why we stray*. New York, NY: Ballantine Books.

Fogel, A. (2009). *The psychophysiology of self-awareness: Rediscovering the lost art of body sense*. New York, NY: W. W. Norton.

Fogel, A., & Garvey, A. (2007). Alive communication, *Infant Behavior & Development, 30*, 251–257.

Fonagy, P., Gergely, G., Jurist, E., & Target, M. (2004). *Affect regulation, mentalization, and the development of the self*. London: Karnac Books.

Fosshage, D. (2011). How do we "know" what we "know?" and change what we "know?" *Psychoanalytic Dialogues, 21*, 55–74.

Franzini, L. (2001). Humor in therapy: The case for training therapists in its uses and risks. *Journal of General Psychology, 128*(2), 170–193.

Frederickson, B. (1998). What good are positive emotions? *Review of General Psychology, 2*(3), 300–319.

Frederickson, B. (2001). The role of positive emotions in positive psychology: The broaden-and-build theory of positive emotions. *American Psychologist, 56*(3), 218–256.

Freeman, W. (1991). The physiology of perception. *Scientific American*, February, 78–85.

Freeman, W. (1999). Consciousness, intentionality, and causality. *Journal of Consciousness Studies, 6*, 143–172.

Freeman, W. (2000). Emotion is essential to all intentional behaviors, In M. Lewis & I. Granic (Eds.), *Emotion, development, and self-organization: Dynamic systems approaches to emotional development* (pp. 209–235). Cambridge, UK: Cambridge University Press.

Gainotti, G. (2012). Unconscious processing of emotion and the right hemisphere. *Neuropsychologia, 50*, 205–218.

Gallese, V. (2001). The "shared manifold" hypothesis: From mirror neurons to empathy. *Journal of Consciousness Studies, 8*(5–7), 33–50.

Gardner, H. (1984). *Art, mind and brain: A cognitive approach to creativity*. New York, NY: Basic Books.

Gazzaniga, M. (2005). Forty-five years of split-brain research and still going strong. *Nature Reviews Neuroscience, 6,* 653–659.

Geller, S., & Greenberg, L. (2002). Therapeutic presence: Therapists' experience of presence in the psychotherapy encounter in psychotherapy. *Person Centered & Experiential Psychotherapies, 1,* 71–86.

Gerrity, P. (1987). Perception in nursing: The value of intuition. *Holistic Nursing Practice, 1*(3), 63–71.

Gilbert, E. (2006). *Eat, pray, love: One woman's search for everything across Italy, India and Indonesia.* New York, NY: Penguin Books.

Gilbert, E. (2009). http://www.ted.com/talks/lang/eng/elizabeth_gilbert_on_genius.html.

Gilligan, C. (1982). *In a different voice: Psychological theory and women's development.* Harvard, MA: Harvard University Press.

Ginot, E. (2009). The empathic power of enactments: The link between neuropsychological processes and an expanded definition of empathy. *Psychoanalytic Psychology, 26*(3), 290–309.

Gladwell, M. (2005). *Blink: The power of thinking without thinking.* New York, NY: Little Brown.

Gladwell, M. (2008). *Outliers: The story of success.* New York, NY: Little, Brown.

Glanz, J. (1997). Mastering the nonlinear brain. *Science, 277,* 1758–1760.

Gleick, J. (1987). *Chaos: Making a new science.* New York, NY: Viking Press.

Goldman, A. (2008). *Simulating minds: The philosophy, psychology and neuroscience of mindreading.* Oxford, UK: Oxford University Press.

Goleman, D. (1997). *Emotional intelligence: Why it can matter more than IQ.* New York, NY: Bantam.

Grastyán, E., Lissák, K., Madarász, I., & Donhogger, H. (1959). Hippocampal electrical activity during the development of conditioned reflexes. *Electroencephalography and Clinical Neurophysiology, 11*(suppl.), 409–430.

Hayles, K. (1990). *Chaos bound: Orderly disorder in contemporary literature and science.* Ithaca, NY: Cornell University Press.

Held, R., & Hein, A. (1963). Movement produced stimulation in the development of visually-guided behavior. *Journal of Comparative and Physiological Psychology, 56*(5), 872–876.

Hershberg, S. (2011). Interfaces between neurobiology, cognitive science, and psychoanalysis: Implicit and explicit processes in therapeutic change. Commentary on papers by Allan N. Schore, Wilma Bucci and James L. Fosshage. *Psychoanalytic Dialogues, 21,* 101–109.

Hillman, J. (1979). *The dream and the underworld.* New York, NY: Harper.

Hirsch, I., & Kessel, P. (1985). Reflections on mature love and transference. *Free Associations, 12,* 60–83.

Hogarth, R. (2001). *Educating intuition.* Chicago, IL: University of Chicago Press.

Hupert, J., Bufka, L., Barlow, D., Gorman, J., Shear, M., & Woods, S. (2001). Therapists, therapist variables, and cognitive-behavioral therapy outcome in a multi-center trial for panic disorder. *Journal of Consulting and Clinical Psychology, 69,* 747–755.

Hynes, C., Baird, A., & Grafton, S. (2006). Differential role of the orbital frontal lobe in emotional versus cognitive perspective-taking. *Neuropsychologia, 44,* 374–383.

Iacoboni, M. (2008). *Mirroring people: The new science of how we connect with others.* New York, NY: Farrar, Straus and Giroux.

Iriki, A. (2006). The neural origins and implications of imitation, mirror neurons and tool use. *Current Opinion in Neurobiology, 16*(6), 660–667.

James, W. (1890). *Principles of psychology* (Vols. 1 & 2). New York, NY: Holt.

Jaušovec, N. (2000). Differences in cognitive processes between gifted, intelligent, creative, and average individuals while solving complex problems: An EEG study. *Intelligence, 28*(3), 213–237.

Kahneman, D. (2002, December 8). *Maps of bounded rationality: A perspective on intuitive judgment and choice.* Nobel Prize lecture, Aula Magna, Stockholm University.

Kalbe, E., Schlegel, M., Sack, A., Nowak, D., Dafotakis, M., Bangard, C., Brand, M., Shamay-Tsoory, S., Onur, O., & Kessler, J. (2010). Dissociating cognitive from affective theory of mind: A TMS study. *Cortex, 26,* 769–780.

Kaslow, F., Cooper, B., & Linsenberg, M. (1979). Family therapist authenticity as a key factor in outcome, *Contemporary Family Therapy, 1*(2), 184–199.

Kestenberg, J. (1985). The flow of empathy and trust between mother and child. In E. Anthony & G. Pollack (Eds.), *Parental influences in health and disease* (pp. 137–163). Boston, MA: Little, Brown.

King, L., & Appleton, J. V. (1997). Intuition: A critical review of the research and rhetoric. *Journal of Advanced Nursing, 26,* 194–202.

Kitzbichler, M., Smith, M, Christensen, S., and Bullmore, E. (2009). Broadband criticality of human brain network synchronization, *PLoS Computational Biology, 5*(3), 1–13.

Knox, J. (2010). *Self-agency in psychotherapy: Attachment, autonomy, and intimacy.* New York, NY: W. W. Norton.

Koestler, A. (1964). *The act of creation.* New York, NY: Macmillan.

Kotler, S. (2010). *A small furry prayer: Dog rescue and the meaning of life.* New York, NY: Bloomsbury.

Kubie, L. (1971). The destructive potential of humor in psychotherapy. *American Journal of Psychiatry, 127,* 861–866.

Kuhl, J., & Kazén, M. (2008). Motivation, affect, and hemispheric asymmetry: Power versus affiliation. *Journal of Personality and Social Psychology, 95*(2), 456–469.

Lakoff, G., & Johnson, M. (1980). *Metaphors we live by.* Chicago, IL: University of Chicago Press.

Lakoff, G., & Johnson, M. (1999). *Philosophy in the flesh: The embodied mind and its challenge to Western thought.* New York, NY: Basic Books.

Lamm, C., Batson, D., & Decety, J. (2007). The neural substrate of human empathy: Effects of perspective-taking and cognitive appraisal. *Journal of Cognitive Neuroscience, 19,* 42–58.

Lamond, D., & Thompson, C. (2000). Intuition and decision making in analysis and choice. *Journal of Nursing Scholarship, 32*(4), 411–414.

Levine, P. (1997). *Healing the tiger: Healing trauma: The innate capacity to transform overwhelming experience.* Berkeley, CA: North Atlantic Books.

Levine, P. (2008). *Healing trauma: A lifelong program for restoring the wisdom of your body.* Louisville, CO: Sounds True Incorporated.

Lewinsohn, P. Mischel, W., Chaplin, W., & Barton, R. (1980). Social competence and depression: The role of illusory self-perceptions. *Journal of Abnormal Psychology, 89*(2), 203–212.

Lewis, J. (2000). Repairing the bond in important relationships: A dynamic for personality maturation, *American Journal of Psychiatry, 157,* 1375–1378.

Lewis, T., Amini, F., & Lannon, R. (2000). *A general theory of love.* New York, NY: Vintage Books.

Libet, B., & Kosslyn, S. (2004). *Mind time: Temporal perspectives in consciousness.* Cambridge, MA: Harvard University Press.

Lieberman, M.D. (2000). Intuition: a social neuroscience approach. *Psychological Bulletin, 126*, 109–137.

Linder, M., Roos, J., & Victor, B. (2001). *Play in organizations*. Working - Paper 2, Imagination Lab Foundation. Retrieved November 10, 2009 from http://www.imagilab.org/research_workingpapers.htm#70

Lutz, W., Leon, S., Martinovich, Z., Lyons, J., & Stiles, W. (2007). Therapist effects in outpatient psychotherapy: A three-level growth curve approach. *Journal of Counseling Psychology, 54*, 32–39.

Lyons-Ruth, K. (1998). Implicit relational knowing: Its role in development and psychoanalytic treatment. *Infant Mental Health Journal, 19*(3), 282–289.

MacLean, P. (1990). *The triune brain in evolution: Role in paleocerebral functioning*. New York, NY: Springer.

MacNeilage, P., Rogers, L., & Vallortigara, G. (2009). Origins of the left and right brain. *Scientific American, 301*(1), 60–67.

Main, M., & Solomon, J. (1990). Procedures for identifying infants as disorganized/disoriented during the Ainsworth Strange Situation. In M. T. Greenberg, D. Cicchetti, & E. M. Cummings (Eds.), *Attachment during the preschool years: Theory, research and intervention* (pp. 121–160). Chicago, IL: University of Chicago Press.

Mancia, M. (2006). Implicit memory and early unrepressed unconscious: Their role in the therapeutic process (How the neurosciences can contribute to psychoanalysis). *International Journal of Psychoanalysis, 87*, 83–103.

Marchetti, V., & Marks, J. (1974). *The CIA and the cult of intelligence*. New York, NY: Knopf.

Marcus, D. M. (1997). On knowing what one knows. *Psychoanalysis Quarterly, 66*, 219–241.

Marks, J. (1979). *The search for the Manchurian candidate*. New York, NY: Times Books.

Marks, J., & Collin Marks, S. (2009). Out of MAD. In C. Stout (Ed.), *The new humanitarians: Inspiration, innovations, and blueprints for visionaries* (pp. 191–212). New York, NY: Praeger.

Marks-Tarlow, T. (1996). *Creativity inside-out: Learning through multiple intelligences*. Palo Alto, CA: Addison-Wesley.

Marks-Tarlow, T. (2003). The certainty of uncertainty. *Psychological Perspectives, 45*, 118–130.

Marks-Tarlow, T. (2008a). *Psyche's veil: Psychotherapy, fractals and complexity*. London: Routledge.

Marks-Tarlow, T. (2008b). Alan Turing meets the sphinx: Some new and old riddles. *Chaos & Complexity Letters, 3*(1), 83–95.

Marks-Tarlow, T (2010). The fractal self at play. *American Journal of Play, 3*(1), 31–62.

Marks-Tarlow, T. (2011). Merging and emerging: A nonlinear portrait of intersubjectivity during psychotherapy. *Psychoanalytic Dialogues, 21*, 110–127.

Marks-Tarlow, T., Robertson, R., & Combs, A. (2002). Varela and the uroboros: The psychological significance of reentry. *Cybernetics & Human Knowing, 9*(2), 31–47.

Mash, E., & Barkley, R. (Eds.). (2003). Child psychopathology (2nd ed.). New York, NY: Guilford.

Maslow, I. (1943). A theory of human motivation. *Psychological Review, 50*, 370–396.

McCrea, S. (2010). Intuition, insight, and the right-hemisphere: Emergence of higher sociocognitive functions. *Psychology Research and Behavior Management, 3*, 1–39.

McGilchrist, I. (2009). *The master and his emissary: The divided brain and the making of the Western world*. New Haven, CT: Yale University Press.

Meares, R. (2005). *The metaphor of play: Origin and break-down of personal being*. London: Routledge.

Meeks, T., & Jeste, D. (2009). Neurobiology of wisdom: A literature review. *Archives of General Psychiatry, 66*(4), 355–365.

Miller, J., Jordan, J., Stiver, I., Walker, M., Surrey, J., & Eldfidge, N. (1999). *Therapists' authenticity: Work in progress* (no. 82). Wellesley, MA: Stone Center Working Paper Series.

Miracle, V. (2007). A personal reflection: Humor—I'd rather laugh than cry. *Dimensions of Critical Care Nursing, 26*(6), 241-243.

Modell, A. (2003). *Imagination and the meaningful brain*. Cambridge, MA: MIT Press.

Moltu, C., Binder, P., & Nielsen, G. (2010). Commitment under pressure: Experienced therapists' inner work during difficult therapeutic impasses. *Psychotherapy Research, 20*(3), 309–320.

Mosak, H. (1987). *Ha ha and aha: The role of humor in psychotherapy*. London: Routledge.

Myers, D. (2002). *Intuition: Its powers and perils*. New Haven, CT: Yale University Press.

Myss, C. (1997). *Anatomy of the spirit: The seven stages of power and healing*. New York, NY: Three Rivers.

Narvaez, D. (2010). Moral complexity: The fatal attraction of truthiness and the importance of mature moral functioning. *Perspectives in Psychological Science, 5*, 163–181.

Natterson, J. (2003). Love in psychotherapy. *Psychoanalytic Psychology, 20*(3), 509–521.

Neihart, M. (2000). Gifted children with Asperger's syndrome. *Gifted Child Quarterly, 44*(4), 222–230.

Nelson, J. (2005). *Seeing through tears: Crying and attachment*. London: Brunner-Routledge.

Newhouse, B. (2008). Examining an amnesiac's brain. *Talk of the Nation* (National Public Radio, NPR). Retrieved December 12, 2008, from http://www.npr.org/templates/story/story.php?storyId=98184825

Nissen-Lie, A., Monsen, J., & Ronnestad, M. (2010). Therapist predictors of early patient-rated working alliance. *Psychotherapy Research, 20*(6), 627–646.

Oakley, B., Knafo, A., Madhavan, G., & Wilson, D. (2011). *Pathological altruism*. New York, NY: Oxford University Press.

Obler, L. & Fein, D. (Eds.). (1988). *The exceptional brain: Neuropsychology of talent and special abilities*. New York, NY: Guilford.

Ogden, P., Minton, K., & Pain, C. (2006). *Trauma and the body: A sensorimotor approach to psychotherapy*. New York, NY: W. W. Norton.

Orloff, J. (2010) *Second sight: An intuitive psychiatrist tells her extraordinary story and shows you how to tap your own inner wisdom*. New York, NY: Three Rivers.

Ostrovsky, Y., Andalman, A., & Sinha, P. (2006). Vision following extended congenital blindness. *Psychological Science, 17*(12), 1009–1014.

Panksepp, J. (1998). *Affective neuroscience: The foundations of human and animal emotions*. New York, NY: Oxford University Press.

Panksepp, J. (2008). Play, ADHD and the construction of the social brain: Should the first class each day be recess? *American Journal of Play, 1*(1), 55–79.

Panksepp, J. (2010). Science of the brain as a gateway to understanding play: Interview with Jaak Panksepp. *American Journal of Play, 2*(3), 245–277.

Panksepp, J. (2011). Cross-species affective neuroscience decoding of the primal affective experiences of humans and related animals. *PLoS ONE, 6*(8), e21236, 1–14.

Panksepp, J. & Watts, D. (2011). Why does depression hurt? Ancestral primary-process separation-distress (PANIC/GRIEF) brain reward (SEEKING) processes in the genesis of depressive affect. *Psychiatry, 74*(1), 5–13.

Pellegrino, E. D. (1979). The anatomy of clinical judgments. Some notes on right reason and right action. In H. T. Engelhardt, S. F. Spicker, & B. Towers (Eds.), *Clinical judgment: A critical appraisal*. Dordrecht, Netherlands: Reidel.

Pellis, S., & Pellis, V. (2010). *The playful brain: Venturing to the limits of neuroscience*. Oxford, UK: Oneworld.

Perrin, W., Würsig, B., & Thewissin, J. (2008). *Encyclopedia of marine biology*. New York, NY: Academic Press.

Piaget, J. (1962). *Play, dreams, and imitation in childhood* (Gattegno, C., & Hodgson, F., Trans.). New York, NY: Norton.

Pincus, D., & Sheikh, A. (2009). *Imagery for pain relief: A scientifically grounded guidebook for clinicians*. New York, NY: Routledge.

Pobric, G., Mashal, N., Faust, M., & Lavidor, M. (2008). The role of the right cerebral hemisphere in processing novel metaphoric expressions: A transcranial magnetic stimulation study. *Journal of Cognitive Neuroscience, 20*(1), 170–181.

Porges, S. (2008). Lecture. Retrieved June, 2009) from http://www.psychevisual.com/Video_by_Stephen_Porges_on_Polyvagal_Theory_1_Basic_principles_p hylogeny_neuroception_dissolution_social_engagement_system.html, Recorded at an invitation by the NSW Service for the Treatment and Rehabilitation of Torture and Trauma Survivors (STARTTS), August 2009, New South Wales, Australia.

Porges, S. (2011). *The polyvagal theory: Neurophysiological foundations of emotions, attachment, communication, and self-regulation*. New York, NY: W. W. Norton.

Prior, V., & Glaser, D. (2006). *Understanding attachment and attachment disorders: Theory, evidence and practice*. Child and Adolescent Mental Health, RCPRTU. London: Jessica Kingsley.

Provine, R. (2000). *Laughter: A scientific investigation*. London: Penguin Books.

Ramachandran, V. (2009), Edge interview, Mirror neurons and imitation learning as the driving force behind "the great leap forward" in human evolution. Retrieved June, 2009 from http://www.edge.org/3rd_culture/ramachandran/ramachandran_index.html

Ramachandran, V. (2004). *A brief tour of human consciousness: BBC Reith lectures*. New York, NY: Pi Press.

Ramachandran, V. (2011). *The tell-tale brain: A neuroscientist's quest for what makes us human*. New York, NY: W. W. Norton.

Reik, T. (1983). *Listening with the third ear*. New York, NY: Farrar, Straus, Giroux.

Rew, L. (1986). Intuition: Concept analysis of a group phenomenon. *Advances in Nursing Science, 8*(2), 21-28.

Rew, L. (1988). Intuition in decision-making. *Journal of Nursing Scholarship, 20*(3), 150–154.

Rew, L., & Barron, E. (1987). Intuition: A neglected hallmark of nursing knowledge. *Advances in Nursing Science, 10*(1), 49–62.

Rizzolatti, G., & Arbib, M. (1998). Language within our grasp. *Trends in Neurosciences, 21*(5), 188–194.

Rose, J. (1984). *The case of "Peter Pan" or, the impossibility of children's fiction*. London: Macmillan.

Rosenblatt, A., & Thickstun, J. (1994). Intuition and consciousness. *Psycho-analytic Quarterly, 63,* 696–714.

Rosanoff, N. (1991). *Intuition workout: A practical guide to discovering and developing your inner knowing.* Fairfield, CT: Aslan.

Rotenberg, V. (2004). The peculiarity of the right-hemisphere function in depression: Solving the paradoxes. *Progress in Neuro-Psychopharmacology & Biological Psychiatry, 28,* 1–13.

Rueckert, L., & Naybar, N. (2008). Gender differences in empathy: The role of the right hemisphere. *Brain and Cognition, 67,* 162–167.

Rustin, J. (1970). Therapist authenticity in group and individual psychother-apy with college students. *Journal of Contemporary Psychotherapy, 3*(1), 45–50.

Ruth-Lyons, K. (2006). Play, precariousness, and the negotiation of shared meaning: A developmental research perspective on child psychotherapy. *Journal of Infant, Child, and Adolescent Psychotherapy, 5*(2), 142–159.

Sands, S. (1984). The use of humor in psychotherapy, *Psychoanalytic Review, 71,* 441–480.

Sands, S. (2011). On the royal road together: The analytic function of dreams in activating dissociative unconscious communication. *Psychoanalytic Dialogues, 20,* 357–373.

Saper, B. (1988). Humor in psychiatric healing, *Psychiatric Quarterly, 59*(4), 306–319.

Sapolsky, R. (1998). *Why zebras don't get ulcers: An updated guide to stress, stress-related diseases and coping.* New York, NY: W. H. Freeman.

Sapolsky, R. (2010, November 14). This is your brain on metaphors. *New York Times.* Retrieved from http://opinionator.blogs.nytimes.com/2010/11/14/this-is-your-brain-on-metaphors/

Schore, A. (1994). *Affect regulation and the origin of the self.* New York, NY: Erlbaum.

Schore, A. (2001). The effects of early relational trauma on right brain dev-elopment, emotional regulation, and infant mental health. *Infant Mental Health Journal, 22*(1–2), 201–269.

Schore, A. (2003a). *Affect dysregulation and disorders of the self.* New York, NY: W. W. Norton.

Schore, A. (2003b). *Affect regulation and the repair of the self.* New York, NY: W. W. Norton.

Schore, A. (2009a). Right-brain affect regulation: An essential mechanism of development, trauma, dissociation, and psychotherapy. In D. Fosha, M. Siegel, & M. Solomon (Eds.), *The healing power of emotion* (pp. 112–144). New York, NY: W. W. Norton.

Schore, A. (2009b). Attachment trauma and the developing right brain: Origins of pathological dissociation. In P. Dell & J. O'Neil (Eds.), *Dissociation and the dis-sociative disorders: DSM-V and beyond* (pp. 107–144). New York, NY: Routledge.

Schore, A. (2010). The right-brain implicit self: A central mechanism of the psychotherapy change process. In J. Petrucelli (Ed.), *Knowing, Not-knowing and sort of knowing: Psychoanalysis and the experience of uncertainty* (pp. 177–202). London: Karnac.

Schore, A. (2011). The right brain implicit self lies at the core of psychoanalytic psychotherapy. *Psychoanalytic Dialogues, 21,* 75–100.

Schore, A. (2012). *The science of the art of psychotherapy.* New York: W.W. Norton.

Schore, J.R., & Schore, A.N. (2008). Modern attachment theory: The central role of affect regulation in development and treatment. *Clinical Social Work Journal, 36,* 9–20.

Schraeder, B., & Fischer, D. (1986). Using intuitive knowledge to make clinical decisions. *American Journal of Maternal/Child Nursing, 11*(3), 161–162.

Schraeder, B., & Fischer, D.K. (1987). Using intuitive knowledge in the neo-natal intensive care nursery. *Holistic Nursing Practice, 1*(3), 45–51.

Searles, H. (1984/1985). The role of the analyst's facial expressions in psycho-analysis and psychoanalytic therapy. *International Journal of Psychoanalysis and Psychotherapy, 10,* 47–73.

Shamay-Tsoory, S., Tomer, R., Berger, B., Goldsher, D., & Aharon-Peretz, J. (2005). Impaired "affective theory of mind" is associated with right ventromedial prefrontal damage. *Cognitive and Behavioral Neurology, 18,* 55–67.

Shaw, D. (2003). On the therapeutic action of therapeutic love. *Contemporary Psychoanalysis, 39*(2), 251–278.

Shedler, J. (2010). The efficacy of psychodynamic psychotherapy. *American Psychologist, 65,* 98–109.

Siegel, D. (1999). *The developing mind: How relationship and the brain interact to shape who we are.* New York, NY: Guilford.

Siegel, D. (2001). Toward an interpersonal neurobiology of the developing mind: Attachment, "mindsight," and neural integration. *Infant Mental Health Journal, 22,* 67–94.

Siegel, D. (2007). *The mindful brain: Reflection and attunement in the culti-vation of well-being.* New York, NY: W. W. Norton.

Siegel, D. (2010). *The mindful therapist: A clinician's guide to mindsight and neural integration.* New York, NY: W. W. Norton.

Siegel, M., & Varley, R. (2002). Neuronal systems involved in "theory of mind." *Nature Reviews, 3,* 463, 471.

Singer, D., & Singer, J. (1990). *The house of make-believe: Children's play and the developing imagination.* Cambridge, MA: Harvard University Press.

Singer, T., Seymour, B., O'Doherty, J., Stephan, K., Dolan, R., & Frith, C. (2006). Empathic neural responses are modulated by the perceived fairness of others. *Nature, 439,* 466–469.

Smilansky, S. (1990). Sociodramatic play: Its relevance to behavior and achieve-ment in school. In E. Klugman & S. Smilansky (Eds.), *Children's play and learn-ing.* New York, NY: Teacher's College.

Snowden, A. (2003). Humor and health promotion. *Health Education Jour-nal, 62*(2), 143–152.

Spencer, H. (1873). *The principles of psychology.* New York, NY: Appleton and Co.

Stern, D. (1985). *The interpersonal world of the infant.* New York, NY: Basic Books.

Stern, D. (2004). *The present moment in psychotherapy and everyday life.* New York, NY: W. W. Norton.

Sternberg, R., & Jordon, J. (2005). *A handbook of wisdom: Psychological per-spectives.* New York, NY: Cambridge University Press.

Stone, M. (2006). The analyst's body as tuning fork: Embodied resonance in countertransference. *Journal of Analytical Psychology, 51,* 109–124.

Strupp, H (1978). The therapist's theoretical orientation: An over-rated vari-able. *Psychotherapy: Theory, Research & Practice, 15*(4), 314–317.

Sutton-Smith, B. (Ed.). (1979). *Play and learning.* New York, NY: Gardner Press.

Sutton-Smith, B. (1997). *The ambiguity of play.* Cambridge, MA: Harvard University Press.

Swain, J. (2011). The human parental brain: In vivo neuroimaging. *Progress in Neuro-Psychopharmacology and Biological Psychiatry, 35*(5), 1242-1254.

Taylor, S., & Brown, J. (1994). Positive illusions and well-being revisited: Separating fact from fiction. *Psychological Bulletin, 116*(1), 21–27.

Thibodeau, L. (2005). *Natural-born intuition: How to awaken and develop your inner wisdom*. Franklin Lakes, NJ: New Page Books.

Thomas, L., De Bellis, M., Graham, R., & LaBar, K. (1997). Development of emotional facial recognition in late childhood and adolescence. *Developmental Science, 10*(5), 547–558.

Trevarthan, C. (2001). Infant intersubjectivity: Research, theory, and clinical applications. *Journal of Child Psychology and Psychiatry, 42*, 3–48.

Tucker, D., Watson, R., & Heilman, K. (1977). Discrimination and evocation of affectively intoned speech in patients with right parietal disease. *Neurology, 27*(10), 947-950.

Tversky, A., & Kahneman, D. (1971). Belief in the law of small numbers. *Psychological Bulletin, 76*, 105–110.

VanderVen, K. (1998). Play, proteus and paradox: Education for a chaotic and supersymmetric world. In D. Pronin & D. Fromberg (Eds.), *Play from birth to twelve and beyond: Contexts, perspectives, and meanings* (pp. 119–132). New York, NY: Garland.

Vanderwolf, C. (1969). Hippocampal electrical activity and voluntary movement in the rat. *Electroencephalography and Clinical Neurophysiology, 26*, 407–418.

Varela, F. (1975). A calculus for self-reference. *International Journal of General Systems, 2*, 5–24.

Varela, F. (1979). *Principles of biological autonomy*. New York, NY: North Holland.

Varela, F., Thompson, E., & Rosch, E. (1991). *The embodied mind: Cognitive science and human experience*. Cambridge, MA: MIT Press.

Vaughan, F. (1979). *Awakening intuition*. New York, NY: Anchor Books.

Vogel, S., Rössler, O., & Marks-Tarlow, T. (2008). *Simultaneity: Temporal structures and observer perspectives*. Singapore: World Scientific.

Volz, K.G., & von Cramon, D.Y. (2006). What neuroscience can tell about intuitive processes in the context of perceptual discovery. *Journal of Cognitive Neuroscience, 18*, 2077–2087.

Vygotsky, L. (1978). Mind in society: The development of higher mental processes (M. Cole, V. John-Steiner, S. Scribner & E. Souberman, Eds. and Trans.). Cambridge, MA: Harvard University Press. (Original work published 1930–1935).

Vygotsky, L. (1986). *Thought and language* (A. Kozulin, Trans.). Cambridge, MA: MIT Press.

Walker, A. (Ed.). (2005). *Understanding quality of life in old age*. New York, NY: Open University Press.

Wampold, B. (2010). The research evidence for common factor models: A historically situated perspective. In B. Duncan, S. Miller, B. Wampold, & M. Hubble (Eds.), *The heart & soul of change: Delivering what works in therapy* (2nd ed., pp. 49-81). Washington, DC: American Psychological Association.

Wampold, B., & Brown, G. (2005). Estimating variability in outcomes attributable to therapists: A naturalistic study of outcomes in managed care. *Journal of Consulting and Clinical Psychology, 73*, 914–923.

Watson, K., Matthews, B., & Allman, J. (2007). Brain activation during sight gags and language-dependent humor. *Cerebral Cortex, 17*(2), 314–324.

Watts, A. (1958). *The wisdom of insecurity*. New York, NY: Pantheon.

Weaver, T., & Clum, G. (1993). Early family environments and traumatic experiences associated with borderline personality disorder, *Journal of Consulting and Clinical Psychology, 61*(6), 1068–1075.

Welling, H. (2005). The intuitive process: The case of psychotherapy, *Journal of Psychotherapy Integration, 15,* 19–47.

White, E. B. (Ed.). (1941). *A subtreasury of American humor*. London: Coward-McCann.

Whitehead, A. (1929). *Process and reality: An essay in cosmology*. New York, NY: Macmillan.

Winnicott, D. W. (1971). *Playing and reality*. New York, NY: Tavistock/Routledge.

Yin, B., & Troger, A. (2011). Exploring the 4th dimention: Hippocampus, time, and memory revisited. *Frontiers in Integrative Neuroscience (www.frontiersin .org), 5,* article 36.

Young, C. (1987). Intuition and nursing process. *Holistic Nursing Practice, 1*(3), 52–62.

Zeanah, C. (Ed.). (2009). *Handbook of infant mental health*. New York, NY: Guilford.

Index

Note: Italicized page locators indicate figures/photos.